STO

ACPL ITEM
DISCARDED

Y0-ABQ-001

* 618 .2 F95H   2193174
FULLER, ELIZABETH, 1946-
HAVING YOUR FIRST BABY
AFTER THIRTY

DO NOT REMOVE
CARDS FROM POCKET

AUG   9 '83

ALLEN COUNTY PUBLIC LIBRARY

FORT WAYNE, INDIANA 46802

You may return this book to any agency, branch,
or bookmobile of the Allen County Public Library.

DEMCO

Having Your First Baby After Thirty

Having Your First Baby After Thirty

A Personal Journey from Infertility to Childbirth

ELIZABETH FULLER

DODD, MEAD & COMPANY
NEW YORK

Copyright © 1983 by Elizabeth Fuller
All rights reserved
No part of this book may be reproduced in any form
without permission in writing from the publisher
Printed in the United States of America

1 2 3 4 5 6 7 8 9 10

Library of Congress Cataloging in Publication Data

Fuller, Elizabeth, 1946–
    Having your first baby after thirty

    Bibliography: p.
    Includes index.
        1. Infertility, Female—Patients—United States—
    Biography.   2. Pregnant women—United States—
    Biography.   3. Fuller, Elizabeth, 1946–
    4. Pregnancy in middle age.   I. Title.
    RG201.F84 1983   618.2 [B]   82-23548
    ISBN 0-396-08154-1

ALLEN COUNTY PUBLIC LIBRARY
FORT WAYNE, INDIANA

To Christopher

2193174

CONTENTS

_____ FOREWORD

Bringing a healthy baby into this world still has to be one of the most joyful and satisfactory experiences of an obstetrician-gynecologist. Not only is there the inevitably close relationship with the mother, and now even the father; but the thought that the pregnancy started out as an egg and sperm cell, each so tiny as to be invisible to the naked eye, and has ended up a completely formed human being is a wondrous thing. However, to a few obstetrics and gynecology practitioners (those who do infertility work) there is an even more joyous and emotional experience. When, after years of frustration and month after month of failure, they place the fetal heart tone detector on the abdomen of a very early infertility patient and hear a definite baby's heartbeat—that has to be an even more exciting moment.

Infertility is a very rewarding experience when you succeed, but a miserable one when you fail. As you will see from Elizabeth's experience, the impact on the psyches of these patients is monumental. But many patients are not aware of the impact on their physician's psyche. Nobody likes month after month of failure; it's not good for anyone's ego. If the nurse says to me that Mrs. X is on the phone to talk to me and she is one of my long-standing nonsuccesses, I realize immediately that she's calling to tell me she got her period again (as we instruct them to do). Sometimes I get so upset that my reaction is: "I don't want to talk to her; you talk to her." It may take me a day or two to get myself together enough to call her, console her, and set up next month's program. Fortunately, I have an extremely capable and sympathetic nurse, and we complement each other. When I am down she is always up and vice versa.

Infertility is a relatively new field of interest. Most of our knowledge has been gained in the last fifty years, and the explosion of knowledge in the last ten years has been incredible. And there is so much we don't know yet. The four major breakthroughs, all within the last ten years, that have dramatically changed women's ability to produce healthy children, have been:

    1.   the ability to induce ovulation with reliable drugs, such as clomiphene citrate and HMG

2. the introduction of microsurgical techniques to repair the damaged or blocked Fallopian tubes and ovaries
3. the use of the laparoscope for more definitive diagnosis
4. the tremendous amount of physiological and chemical knowledge we have gained and will continue to glean from *in vitro* fertilization techniques.

Advances we can look forward to are:

1. the ability to influence formation of the sperm as we now can influence the ovary
2. the elucidation of the many physico-chemical changes that occur within the Fallopian tube to the sperm, egg, and fertilized ovum as they pass through
3. an understanding of the role of environmental influences on the achievement of pregnancy.

The next ten years should be extremely rewarding ones for the future of infertility, but probably one thing that will never change is the impact infertility has on the interpersonal relationships of wife, husband, friends, and physician, as beautifully told here by Elizabeth Fuller.

Robert L. Madison, M.D.
Associate Chief of Obstetrics
and Gynecology, Stamford
Hospital

1

The Fertility Workup

At five years old, I dragged my Tiny Tears doll around, dreaming of the day I'd be a card-carrying mother. At ten years old, I pitched Tiny Tears, got a pair of Mickey Mouse ears and dreamed of being a Mousketeer. At fifteen, the ears and tears were long gone. My fantasies had matured. Now I wanted to become a stewardess and get as far away from Cleveland Heights as possible—perhaps all the way to Chicago. At twenty, I got my wings and moved to Minneapolis. For once a dream had finally materialized.

Seven years later, I met my match. Of course I had to go through one short-term marriage before meeting the "Real Thing." At twenty-eight the Real Thing and I got married. He was a journalist and I was his assistant. We traveled all over the world. At thirty I became a writer too, with the publication of my first book. The future held nothing but the promise of excitement, adventure, and intellectual stimulation.

But then at thirty-two something happened. It was as if my inner computer had gone haywire. I became obsessed again with those dreams I had had at the age of five. I wanted nothing more than to trade in the travel, the excitement, and the stimulation in favor of the kind of life style that turns human beings into robots for squealing, squalking baby monsters.

I don't know why this hit so suddenly and with so little warning. Perhaps it had something to do with a biological need that is programmed into all women, though I've known plenty of women who have chosen never to have children who certainly haven't lost sleep over any unfulfilled biological urge. In fact, it appeared to be quite the opposite. My friend Barbara, for example, had a successful career as a C.P.A. for a large New York firm, was happily married, had few financial concerns and lots of free time to have two-hour lunches.

One day, while we were having one of those lunches, an extra glass of Chablis prompted me to confide in her. I told her that I'd like to have a baby. As soon as I had said it, I wished I hadn't. Without mincing words, she told me exactly how she felt about motherhood. She said that I was not only a cop-out to myself, but to all aware women. Over dessert she got into zero population growth.

I couldn't simply dismiss Barbara's views. They were all valid. And at the time I had no well thought out argument as to why I would even remotely consider motherhood. I just had a few points, like what would happen if in ten years I woke up and regretted never having had a child? For which Barbara came back with, "What if in ten years you wake up and realize you hate kids?"

I tried pointing out to Barbara how everything in life is a gamble. Even she was taking a chance that in ten years she would still enjoy accounting. Barbara said merely that if and when she no longer liked her job she would simply leave the firm. But what would I do if I didn't like motherhood—leave the house?

Then Barbara reminded me that only months earlier I had told her how happy and fulfilled I was with my own writing. For the first time in my life I had had a sense of real accomplishment. And now she warned that I was going to go and blow it all on a vacuous whim—a whim that could turn me into a homemaking turnip.

By that evening I had put our luncheon discussion out of my mind. I had other more important things to deal with. The first concerned my husband. He had been married before and had three grown children. One thing I was certain of: he wanted nothing to do with babies—ours or anyone else's. The only time John and I ever discussed babies was after one of my friends dropped by with her kids. John and I both agreed that nothing ruined a good time quicker than a kid. In fact I had lost a close friend because I had once asked her if she would mind getting a sitter for her two small children. I qualified this by telling her that it wasn't me who minded the kids, it was John. He claimed that any creature under two feet tall made him nervous. But the truth of the matter was, I didn't like them running around getting their gummy little hands all over everything any more than John did.

John and I often talked about how lucky we were. Our relationship wasn't based on any neurotic need to populate the world. More than once John had said that he had always dreamed of finding a woman like me— one he could work side-by-side and travel with, one who had her own interests.

Now I had a problem. I had no idea how I would break it to John that the woman he had always dreamed of finding would suddenly want to turn into what Barbara called a "homemaking turnip." And the husband problem was just the beginning. During the next three years I was to go through two dozen temperature charts, four basal thermometers, one operation, a postcoital exam, fifty-four visits to a fertility specialist, and hundreds of whimpering telephone calls to close friends. I also went through a few now not-so-good friends because, in their words, I became an unbearable bore.

But bore or no bore, I could not control my sudden compulsive behavior. The only thing I could possibly blame it on was that deep maternal instinct that surfaced at about the same time as a few stray gray hairs and faint bird lines underneath the lower lashes.

In retrospect, the first thing I should have done when the urge hit was to level with my husband. I could have told him that I had never intended to spring such a surprise on him. And that at the time we got married I had never given having a child a thought—not a positive thought anyway. But that now I felt that if I didn't have a baby I would never be a complete human being.

But I didn't do that. After many hours of soul searching I came to the conclusion that there was a distinct possibility that he'd say, flat out, "No baby," and that I could not accept. I was afraid that his thing against babies was bigger than the two of us. I didn't think that it was something that we could sit down and rationally discuss.

What I did do was resort to what he later called "slippery and without principle." I simply and silently went off my birth control pills.

Theoretically, this should have worked, since 65 percent of women who go off the pill conceive within the first six months. But six months later there was no sign of pregnancy.

About four months after I had gone off the pill, I was watching an early morning talk show on which a gynecologist from a New York fertility clinic was discussing infertility and the special problems associated with an "elderly primapara," a woman over thirty-five having her first child.

I felt as if this doctor were talking directly to me. He said that often a woman puts off having a family until she has built a career. But after thirty, she suddenly feels an overwhelming desire to have a baby. This desire, he said, is too frequently complicated by the fact that she feels as if her time is running out. That was me. Every time I got my period I felt one month closer to the Geritol set. He even mentioned something about well-meaning family and friends who usually help confirm these ungrounded fears. That was another thing I could relate to. My mother stopped dropping hints about babies when I turned thirty. It was as if I had suddenly dried up and turned into a fig. The other relatives weren't as subtle. The only person who never commented was my father. I think his fear was that I'd have a baby and drop it off for a three-month visit while John and I went trekking in the Himalayas.

The doctor went on to say that although female fertility does decline after thirty-five, it is not as low as was once believed. With the recent advances in the treatment of infertility and with proper prenatal care, most women over thirty-five can safely have a baby. But then he added that a woman in her thirties who has been trying to conceive for six months unsuccessfully should not wait the usual year to seek fertility counseling. She and her partner should see a specialist after six months.

Perhaps I suspected something might be wrong, because I jotted the clinic's telephone number down. Two months later I phoned the clinic, explained my problem, and was put in touch with a specialist in the area.

Three weeks after that I sat in the specialist's waiting room looking around at the other patients. Several of them seemed as if they were right out of high school. I quickly ruled out their having any fertility problems. It was probably the other way around. Sitting close to me were two women who looked about my age and who must have been used to the long wait. They weren't gaping at others the way I was. In fact, the one sitting next to me was studying some sort of chart with the same intensity as the woman across from her was reading *Baby Talk* magazine. At the opposite end of the room I noticed a woman who looked several years older than me. I pegged her as a regular, because she was joking with the nurses and calling them by name. I was wondering whether she was there to have a baby, and if so, whether she wanted one as badly as I did. For some reason, I felt as if I could relate to her. I suddenly wanted to get up, go over to her, and pour my heart out. But of course I didn't.

Ever since I made the decision to get pregnant, my emotions had been running the gamut from ecstasy at the thought of having a baby to depression at the thought of never having one—and deep depression when I thought that I was doing this behind my husband's back. For up until that time, John and I had had no secrets. That had been one of the best things about our marriage. Now this obsession with having a baby threatened to undermine the best thing I had ever had.

But I couldn't stop myself. It was as if I were possessed. Intellectually, I knew that our life style could never include a baby. We spent at least three months a year traveling to remote parts of the world on research. On top of that, I should have felt satisfied. I had written and published two books and was working on a third— not that either one of them had become a household word, but I did feel a great sense of accomplishment. Had I not felt this way, I could have understood why I so desperately wanted a baby. The only thing I had to go on was that maternal instinct. There were times I went to sleep praying that I'd wake up and this crazy obsession would be gone. But there were other times when I seemed to enjoy wallowing in my misery. I was just starting to slide into that wallowing mood when the nurse appeared at the door and called my name.

I felt as if I had been kept waiting in the icy examining room two days, but my watch said it had been only fifteen minutes. When the doctor finally entered, I was reassured: he looked young enough to know all the latest fertility techniques and old enough to have had on-the-job experience.

The first thing he did was to take the usual medical history. I had gone through this many times as part of my annual checkup. Following that, he did a pelvic exam. After he completed the exam, he told me to get dressed and meet him in his office. So far I had found out nothing about myself. I did, however, learn that he had just returned from a two-week sailing trip during which it rained almost every day.

But once inside his office he explained that, although my pelvic exam appeared normal, that was only the very first step in what would be a three-month basic preliminary "workup." With that, he scribbled the four steps of the workup on a prescription pad and passed it across his desk. It read: Step 1. temperature charts; Step 2. postcoital (2–3); Step 3. hysterosalpingogram (X-ray of the uterus); Step 4. laparoscopy (hospital).

Before he told me exactly what it was I was reading, he took an additional and more detailed medical and menstrual history, asking when I first began menstruating, how long the bleeding lasted, whether or not my periods were painful. He asked: Is there ever an obvious change in the flow? What types of birth control have I used? How long had I been on the pill? Have I had any abortions? What about miscarriages? Have I ever had a venereal disease? How often did I have sex? When did I have sex? In what position did I have sex? Is intercourse painful?

Even though I like to think of myself as a mature person, I had a hard time answering the last few questions. I'm a typical product of the "Catholic school syndrome" of the fifties and sixties: anything even remotely connected with sex could cause lateral nystagmus, a rapid uncontrollable movement of the eye.

After a barrage of questions, the doctor got into my husband's sexual history. The first thing he wanted to know was his age. I was afraid he was going to ask that. I told him that nobody would ever take John for a day over fifty, and that when I had first met him four years earlier, I could have sworn he was only in his late forties. And that even people who have known him for years can't believe how young he looks.

I couldn't be sure if the doctor was taking it all in. He just sat there tapping a silver pen on his thick oak desk. Finally he smiled and said, "Sounds like a tennis player." Then he leaned back and added, "But Mrs. Fuller, I must know his chronological age. You see, it's a very important part in the workup."

When I told him that John was sixty-five, he immediately stopped tapping the pen. He sat up straight, methodically lowered his wire rims, peered over them, and said that he would like to see a sperm count. I asked if that was because of his age. Without answering me directly, he said that a sperm count is always the first part of a basic preliminary workup for a male of any age. Fertility, he said, is a two-way street. The male must receive as thorough an examination as the female. However, he qualified this by saying that recent statistics on infertility indicate that the male is responsible for roughly 30 to 40 percent of the problems and the female for 60 to 70 percent. That, he said, was because the female has more working parts that can malfunction.

Before I had a chance to ask whether my husband's age could be a big factor in my infertility, he enthusiastically told me that he had seen some pro-football players with a sperm count of as low as 5 million per milliliter, and some octagenarians with a count of 60 million per milliliter. He reminded me that Charlie Chaplin had a baby at eighty. I liked this doctor right away. He was an optimist.

He continued to record my husband's medical history. Finally he took out a sheet of paper with instructions for a sperm count and suggested that the sooner my husband had the count the quicker we could eliminate one potential problem. I knew at that point I'd have to come out of the closet with my secret.

I was praying that if there was a fertility problem it lay with me, not John. I had read in more than one book that when a male's fertility is questioned it is a serious blow to his ego. Even intelligent men confuse infertility with impotence.

As the doctor handed me the instruction sheet for John he asked, "What does your husband think about starting a family at his age?"

I didn't think it was quite the time to confess that my husband was unaware of my efforts to have a baby. I just answered by saying that my husband had three children, and was an excellent father. That finished off all discussion of my husband, and we got back to me.

This time the doctor reached around behind his desk to a small, low table and brought out a two-foot, see-through plastic model of a woman's body. It showed the reproductive organs in living color. Although I had seen plexiglass models in high school biology, I was never exactly sure what went where.

With his silver pointer in hand, he went on to say that the first thing there has to be for conception to occur is an adequate number of healthy sperm deposited deep into the vagina. The vagina is a narrow elastic canal about four to five inches long connected to the cervix, the entrance to the uterus. Since the vagina is acidic and the sperm alkaline, the sperm have to get out of the vagina and into the uterus quickly before they are killed off by the vagina's acidity. For this to be possible the cervical mucous has to have just the right consistency. It must be thin and penetrable. This happens only once a month, at the time of ovulation. During the rest of the month the cervical mucous is thick and impassable and acts as a barrier, preventing the sperm from getting through to the uterus.

It is not enough for the sperm merely to get inside the uterus, however. The uterus must be normal. It must be the size and shape of a hollow, upside-down pear. At the top of the uterus and off to each side is a tiny duct leading into the Fallopian tube, the tube that transports the egg to the uterus.

Meanwhile, an ovary must have created a mature egg, a process called "ovulation." A woman is born with all her eggs—some four hundred thousand of them. And she has two ovaries, each the size and shape of a walnut, one on each side of the uterus, just off the Fallopian tubes. Approximately fourteen days after the menstrual flow, one of these eggs will ripen and pop out of the surface of one of the ovaries. The ovaries generally alternate from month to month. However, if a woman has only one ovary, it will do double the work load.

Once the egg has left the ovary, it begins the journey down the Fallopian tube. The Fallopian tubes start at the top of the uterus on each side and widen like trumpets to open into the abdominal cavity. The egg is helped through the Fallopian tube by little hairlike structures called cilia. This tube is only four to four and a half inches long, with the inside diameter about the width of a broom straw. The egg, although the largest cell in the female body, is only one-fourth the size of the period at the end of this sentence, barely visible to the naked eye. It lives only twelve to twenty-four hours. If the egg hasn't hooked up with a sperm in that length of time, it's finished and is shed in the next menstrual flow.

But if the healthy sperm have made that long swim upstream into the Fallopian tube, it's a whole different story. Only a few sperm out of a possible one hundred to three hundred million that are released in each ejaculation need penetrate the egg's smooth shell. And of those only one will actually fertilize the egg. Once the egg has been fertilized, it begins to divide while continuing to travel the rest of the way down the tube—a process that takes several days—and finally implants in the wall of the uterus where the lining has been developed properly. The uterus will house the newly fertilized egg for the next nine months if all goes well. At the end of the nine months, the uterus will have expanded from the size of the pear to forty times its normal nonpregnant state. But conception will only happen if the conditions are absolutely perfect.

Now the doctor began elaborating on some of the more common things that can go wrong. He said that one of the major causes of infertility after the age of thirty is a condition known as endometriosis. This occurs when part of the normal uterine lining appears outside the uterus in areas such as the tubes, ovaries, or the surface of the abdominal cavity. Women who have had babies before the age of thirty usually don't have this trouble. Part of the reason is that the cervix has dilated. With a dilated cervix it is much easier for the menstruation blood to come out of the cervix and vagina. There is less pressure, so it doesn't back up through the tubes. It is backed-up blood that causes the misplaced endometrium. And this endometrium will respond to a woman's hormones the same way her uterine tissue responds. It, too, will bleed at the time of her period, resulting in the scarring, adhesions, and cysts that develop on her pelvic organs. It also causes severe pain during menstruation. I guessed that that was why the doctor asked me if I had painful periods. I told him that I didn't.

He went on to say that, strangely enough, women who have been on the pill for many years seem to have a much smaller chance of getting endometriosis. They bleed less, so there is less tissue inside the uterus that has to come out, less of a chance of the tissue backing up through the cervix into the tubes, causing the scarring and adhesions. In fact, one of the nonsurgical treatments is to put a woman on the pill with no monthly interruption for eight or nine months to stop her periods, creating a pseudopregnancy. Once her periods are stopped the misplaced endometrium will die.

As the doctor was tapping that silver pen against the plastic model's ovaries, Fallopian tubes, cervix, and uterus, I suddenly recalled all the months of tension, all the months of keeping my obsession inside. Except for

Barbara, I had told no one. Suddenly all the hope I had of having a baby seemed wasted, all the fears that I might *never* have one welled up. I started to cry.

I felt like such a fool. I was no longer in control. I usually cover my emotions with a sense of humor, but now I couldn't think of anything funny to say. Because there wasn't anything funny. I wanted a baby and suddenly I was face to face with all these possibilities that might stop me from getting what I wanted. I felt angry. I felt sorry for myself. I felt deserving. I felt undeserving. I felt confused. I was crying, and I really didn't know why. I didn't know if my tears were legitimate. Did I want the doctor to feel sorry for me? Did I want attention? Did I want him to say, as my parents always did, that I shouldn't worry—it'll all work out?

He must have been used to this. He wasted no time sliding a box of tissues my way. But he still didn't say anything. I thought that this is what it must be like to go to a shrink. Finally he began to console me by describing all the modern techniques available to deal with infertility. But I wasn't listening. I didn't want to know about laparoscopes or hysterosalpingograms. I wanted to know about those young girls sitting in the waiting room. Were they there to have babies? Were their chances twice as good as mine? And what about the older woman who was joking with the nurses? Was she there to have a baby? Would I end up in five years like her, joking instead of crying? And what about the other lady sitting next to me poring over some temperature chart as if it were a matter of life and death? Would I be doing that month after month? And what about the lady across from her who was reading *Baby Talk?* Would I be sitting there making myself sicker reading about how to bathe your baby in safety and comfort while pregnant women marched in and out of the office? And if I was going to end up like that I wanted to know. And I wanted to know right away.

But the rational side of me knew better than to ask such questions. They were unreasonable. So I said nothing. Instead I silently nodded my head as he explained that the first step in my workup—a phrase that still made me feel as if I were going in for a lube job—would be to keep a temperature chart. The idea behind the chart was to see if I was ovulating.

Every morning, before I got out of bed or before I did anything to even slightly raise my body temperature, I would place a basal thermometer in my mouth for five minutes. After I got a temperature reading, I would then record it on the chart next to the day of my cycle. The first day of bleeding is called day 1. If I am ovulating, the temperature graph plotted during the twenty-eight-day cycle should show a slight midcycle temperature drop of one-half to one degree. The twenty-four hours following this drop in temperature is the period immediately following ovulation.

That, the doctor said, is considered the best time to get pregnant. I would be at my maximum fertility and should have intercourse on days 11, 13, 15, and 17 of my cycle. As if this weren't regimented enough, he told me not to forget to draw a circle around the temperature mark on the day we had intercourse.

I knew this was necessary, but it was still people breeding. All of this reminded me of the time I took my female beagle to meet her match. The lady who bred her was so matter-of-fact about what I thought should have been a very sensitive issue that I almost grabbed my beagle and split. Now that I think about it, she and the doctor used similar jargon. They both said "maximum fertility" a lot, although she threw around words like *heat, bitch,* and *mate,* while he threw around *ovulation, woman,* and *intercourse.* The tone of the discussion was in the same vein. I remember mentioning to the dog lady how cut and dry it all seemed. She looked at me as if I were certifiable, and told me plain out that she didn't do music, wine, or candles.

I left the doctor's office that day with a three-month supply of temperature charts in one hand and an appointment slip for a month later in the other. Once I got out to the parking lot, I decided that I couldn't go right home. I needed time to think. I needed time to figure out the best way to approach John, or whether I would approach him at all. What I needed was advice. But not the kind of advice Barbara would give me.

This time I picked a friend who was a little more maternally oriented than Barbara. Her name was Patsy. We had met one evening at a party shortly after she, her husband, and their three children moved from London to Connecticut. Although our experiences were vastly different, we did share one common interest: art. In fact the night we met, I told her all about my art class, how fulfilling and rewarding it was. I even liked her enough to confide in her how a well-known artist in the area took one look at my canvases and only half-jokingly said that I'd be just as well off in a home-study paint-by-numbers course. The following week Patsy joined the class. I guess she felt I was no threat.

Now a year after we had met, and thirty minutes after I had left the doctor's office, she greeted me at the door, looking as if she had just stepped out of a drain pipe. But in spite of the red scarf around her head, the rubber gloves, and the drenched sweat pants hiked up as if for a flood, she looked graceful. Up until she turned thirty, she had been a professional ballet and modern dancer on the London stage. Now at forty and three kids later, she still looked thirty and as if at any moment she was going to spring a *grande jeté.*

Patsy led me into the bathroom, and instructed her golden lab, Sam, to hop back into the tub. As she soaped and sudsed Sam, I spilled my guts out. I told her the whole story from the time I first got the urge to have a baby up until the present. In fact it wasn't until I began talking that I realized just when this desire to have a child had hit. It went back almost a year to the time my husband and I were researching a book in the Himalayas.

John and I were trekking at fourteen thousand feet when our Sherpa guides spotted a three-year-old boy who had just fallen into an open-pitted fire. We cleaned the child up, applied what first aid we had, gave him a chocolate bar and a week's worth of rupees, and sent him home to his mother. But our guides learned that he had no mother. He was an orphan. When I heard that, I insisted that we take him with us, even though we were headed toward Mount Everest. Our guides wouldn't hear of it. They were right. They explained that the boy was from that village and that the villagers made sure he was fed and had a place to sleep at night. If we took him to a strange village, he would be stranded.

For months I was haunted by the image of the shoeless little boy in some sort of ragged brown sack cloth, crying after us. I was angry at myself for not having insisted that we do more for him. I thought maybe there was some way John and I could have adopted him. The only thing I knew about the child was that his mother had fled to the lowlands with a new husband, and his father had just skipped out. I didn't know his mother or father, but I hated them anyway. How could they leave their child? It was at that point I thought to myself: if I couldn't have that child, I'd have my own. This was twisted and confused thinking. How could *my* having a child possibly make up for *that* child's miserable life?

Although we never brought back that shoeless little boy, we did bring back another. His name was Nima. He was our eighteen-year-old Sherpa guide who had two dreams—to see the world, and then to build a teahouse. He told us about the teahouse when he showed us the logs he had cut and stored near his house, which sat practically in the shadow of Mount Everest. His teahouse would be a small, elongated cabin with a cozy fire in an open pit, a few rough-hewn tables and benches, illuminated by burning yak butter in bronze bowls. There would be two or three bunk rooms for yak-caravan traders or European trekkers who came in from the strong winds that swept down from Everest.

But John and I knew that this dream teahouse was doomed. Nima was in the advanced stages of tuberculosis and he needed prompt medical attention. Since there was no real treatment for T.B. in Nepal, we arranged for Nima to visit us in the United States.

Nima's six-month visit turned out to be a success. He slowly went from 85 pounds to 135. Within weeks his strength returned.

Nima's parting was as difficult for him as it was for us. We had grown to love Nima as if he were our son. And Nima grew to love us. He would often say, "Memsahib same like mother. Sahib like father. Nima like son."

But that was months earlier and Nima was gone. I felt a vacancy. It was like losing a son. I told Patsy that that may have been one reason why I now had to have my own child.

After I finished telling Patsy my story, we all moved from the bathroom to the kitchen where Sam ate, Patsy cooked, and I continued my month-by-month analysis of why I thought I was driven to have a baby. Except for a few kids tearing in and out, I had her undivided attention. But I guess I must have started repeating myself, because Patsy finally interrupted. And when she did, she gave my dilemma a whole new perspective.

Up until this time I had expected to find just one reason why I so desperately wanted a baby. But as Patsy pointed out, there is no *one* reason. There is a lifetime of reasons. It didn't start with the Tiny Tears doll or with the little Himalayan boy. And there were nearly thirty years of reasons in between. She was right. It was suddenly all so obvious. It wasn't just because I wanted to experience pregnancy and childbirth. Or because I always just assumed I'd grow up and have a baby. Or because women were supposed to have babies. Or because I was curious as to what my baby would look and act like. Or because I wanted a child who could make up for all the things I didn't do. Or because I didn't want to be left alone in my old age. It was all of those reasons. Nobody has a baby for just *one* reason.

She also helped allay my fears that, if I did have a child, I would cease to be a functioning human being. I wouldn't have to sit around glued to television soap operas as I lobbed Fig Newtons into a Port-A-Crib to shut the kid up. No, I wouldn't have to be a slave to a baby. As Patsy said, "No eight-pound infant with the I.Q. of a rattle has ever dictated what his mother can or can't do. *You* make yourself into a babbling idiot."

Again she was right. We all make our own choices. The only thing Patsy didn't have any advice on was how I should break this whole thing to John. All she said was, "Darling, I think it's immaterial whether John wants a baby or not." I guess what she meant was that I was going to have a baby and that was that. On my way out she said, "And, Lizzy, when you do have that little bundle of joy, no dump-offs here."

2

Temperature Charts

It was three months after my visit to Patsy, and I still hadn't told John about his required fertility test—or about anything to do with a baby. I blamed Patsy for that. Each time I was about to break the news to him, her words skipped through my mind: "Darling, I think it's immaterial whether John wants a baby or not." I figured that since I was going to have a baby anyway, there was no use upsetting him—at least not until I found out whether or not I was ovulating.

During those three months, I made two more trips to the doctor's office, each month bringing with me a meticulously recorded temperature chart. It was a good

23

thing John felt a neurotic need to get up at five o'clock every morning to write. Otherwise, he surely would have noticed my suspicious behavior with the basal thermometer. I must admit that after I got the hang of using the instrument, it became like a game of Lotto. I used to bet with myself what my temperature would register. If I came within a tenth of a degree, I would treat myself to an extra fifteen minutes in the sack.

My efforts at keeping those charts paid off. The doctor said that, according to my midcycle temperature drop, then sharp rise, I was ovulating. But now he wanted to know why three months had gone by and John still hadn't had a sperm count. I made some lame excuse. I told him that John had been busy meeting deadlines. I think the doctor smelled a rat. He just said that he understood how difficult something like this was, especially for a male. But we still could go no further in the workup without the test.

Since I had no intention of stopping the workup, I had no choice but to go home with the news. And the best time for a news flash would be at dinner, when John would be most receptive to new ideas.

I could not have ordered a more perfect evening. I was almost tempted to say nothing. But the doctor's words persisted: "We can go no further in the workup without your husband's sperm count." I had no choice but to take advantage of John's good mood. First I took a sip of wine, then a deep breath.

"I want to have a baby," I said.

Naturally the first thing that popped into his suspicious head was that I was already pregnant. When I reassured him that I wasn't, he breathed a sigh of relief and said that I had almost given him a heart attack. In the future I was to please not startle him that way again. Then he went on to say that the minute he walked in and saw the candles and the bottle of wine with a cork instead of a screw-on cap, he knew I was up to something.

John's reaction was not one I had hoped for. But I wasn't angry and I wasn't hurt. In fact, if anything, I felt as if I deserved to feel rotten. Here was the man I loved more than anything. And here I was, about to wreck his life. But I couldn't indulge myself in this type of thinking. If I did, I would never finish telling him the entire saga of the past nine months.

"I've been off the pill for nearly a year," I said.

John was no longer comfortably sprawled on the sofa. He was propped up against one of our barn-wood posts. "You've been off the pill? Behind my back?"

I tried to explain how I had had no choice. But he wouldn't listen. He just kept repeating something about when people decide to have a baby they talk about it, they discuss it, they don't slip off and do sneaky things.

I told John that if I really wanted to be sneaky, I wouldn't be telling him about it now. But then he asked the obvious. Why *was* I telling him now? I was left with no choice but to tell him why.

"Because," I said, "there's a very critical, essential process involved."

"Like consulting your husband?" he asked.

"More or less. That's sort of a good description."

"And how many others have you consulted before you let me in on it?"

"Just one other person." I couldn't tell him that I had already told Barbara and Patsy, so I thought I'd just tell him that it was the doctor, for the moment anyway.

"And that's your friend Patsy."

"No. It's not Patsy," I said, "it's the gynecologist."

"You mean that some creepy doctor is standing over your shoulder, telling us how to run our lives?"

I didn't mind that John overreacted as much as I minded the way he just stared at me after every word. This direct eye contact made me feel criminal. I tried telling him that I was driven. That I loved him. That I wanted to have a child of his. That I've never had a child. That I wanted one so badly. I even pulled out that shoeless little Himalayan boy and the Nima story to strengthen my case. But those same stories that had choked Patsy up had little effect on John.

"Liz," John said, "it's out of the question. When I drive the kid to college, I'll be eighty-five years old!" Then John really got dramatic. He began pacing up and down our living room, modulating each word. "And that's the good news. Because it got worse. No peace. No quiet. No travel. No . . ."

"You're overreacting," I said.

"Overreacting? I'm not a businessman. I can't retire at sixty-five. I don't have any big bonus, separation pay, a fat pension. I have to keep going."

"Maybe that's what keeps you young."

"Deadlines don't keep anybody young. They're murderous. Can you imagine meeting a deadline with a little rug rat tugging at my typewriter ribbon? There's just no two ways about it. Old writers can't have babies!"

John went on protesting. He dragged in every reason why we couldn't have a baby, ranging from the macabre to the ludicrous. Somehow I had expected this reaction. I sat mutely, half listening, half lost in my own thoughts. The worst part about what he was saying was that it was all true. And everything I had to say in my defense was all wrong. John said we couldn't have a baby because of the money, research travel, his age. I said I wanted a baby because I loved him, I had never had a child, and I was driven.

As John rambled on with a confident annoying rasp in his voice, something inside of me clicked. I thought: why should his unemotional, logical reasons be any more valid than mine? What was wrong with wanting a baby just because I wanted one? Where was it written that I had to list ten practical reasons for having a baby? Then Patsy's words came back to me: "Lizzy, why are you always looking for reasons?"

She was right. Why couldn't I accept the fact that there are a lifetime of reasons and leave it at that? Why did I have to pinpoint everything I did? Why wasn't it legitimate for me to be in touch with my own emotions? And now, why was I letting John intimidate me with his tangible, practical reasons? Were men programmed to do this to women? And were women programmed to let them get away with it? But John wasn't like most men—at least he hadn't been up until now.

The more I thought about it, the more I was convinced that my reasons were as valid as his. I began to feel sorry for myself—sorry that I ever got myself into a situation where I had to defend a basic human right. Suddenly I felt the same way I had felt three months before, sitting in the doctor's office and watching him poke at the plastic model's reproductive system, telling me of all the physical things that could prevent me from having a baby. Now it was John's turn. He was telling me all the practical considerations that were preventing me from having a baby. I sensed a conspiracy.

As John continued his sales talk, I sat there smoldering.

"*Please* don't look at me like that," he said. "You know how that Neanderthal stare of yours affects me."

That was when I told him how his insensitivity affected me. I was being denied the opportunity to fulfill my maternal urge, and I believed no human being had the right to deny another that basic right. I went on to say that I couldn't even begin to imagine what my life would be like without a baby. The issue was bigger than the two of us. I forget what else I said, but whatever it was, he finally said, "You've apparently got your heart and mind set on a baby."

"You mean," I said, "you'll go along with it?"

"Have I a choice?"

I was so relieved that I think I began to rush things a little. I immediately went over to my handbag and took out the temperature charts that I had brought back from the doctor's office only hours earlier.

"I've got to show you something," I said, resting the charts on his lap.

He studied them for a few seconds, then asked, "What are these?"

Before I had a chance to explain, he began to read aloud the instructions that were printed on the bottom of one of the charts.

" 'Daily Basal Temperature Ovulation Chart. Please indicate days when intercourse takes place by drawing a circle around the daily temperature mark.' " He dropped the charts on his lap and said, "This is so damn clinical!"

"John. It's important!"

"You've been hiding this from me for three months?"

"See all those circles?" I asked. "Aren't you proud?"

But from John's body language I could tell that he wasn't proud. "That damn doctor of yours has been looking over my shoulder for three months!"

I tried changing the subject to something a little more positive. "You notice," I said, "the only time the circles fall off is when you're facing a deadline. I pointed that out to the doctor. I explained it."

"Who does he think he is—God?"

"He's helping us," I said.

"Look, my books get reviewed and edited, but this is too much."

Again I tried focusing on the positive. "The only

time you were a little shaky was this past week. With all the pressure. Otherwise, he was very proud of you."

"*He* was proud of *me!* *He* was proud of *me!*" John was almost shouting. "Elizabeth, how can you do this? It's so cold-blooded." Then he studied the charts again and asked, "And on top of this—why *haven't* we had a baby? I've been doing pretty damn well at my age!"

I explained that that was the very reason we had to find out more about us. And that the doctor said that, although we had been doing very well on the outside, we didn't exactly know what was going on inside.

"What are you getting at, Liz?"

It was then I explained to John what my doctor had told me. That the sperm count, regardless of the man's age, or if he's had previous children, was the first thing to be checked in the male's workup. I kept stressing that I was *sure* that the problem lay with me, not him. Finally John tossed the temperature chart onto the coffee table, sighed loudly, and said that he would go along with having the test. What was he supposed to do?

Before he had a chance to change his mind, I went back to my handbag and got out the instruction sheet that my doctor had given me to give to John. It spelled out the exact procedure for a semen analysis.

1. Patient should abstain from relations for two to three days before test.
2. Specimen is collected by masturbating into a clean, dry container (available from the office if needed)

and brought to the office within two hours after collection.

3. Keep the specimen container in coat or jacket pocket from the time of collection until it is brought to the office to prevent it from becoming cold.

4. On the container the following information should be recorded: name of patient and wife. Time of collection.

John looked up from the mimeographed sheet.

"This," he said, "is the most effective way anyone could possibly devise to take the complete joy out of sex!" Then he added with sarcasm, "But it's nice to be married to such a thorough researcher. So what happens after I follow the instructions?"

He was right. I am a thorough researcher.

The following day, I went through a few infertility books at the library and found out exactly what happened.

Once the sample has been collected, it must be examined in the laboratory, within two to four hours for optimum results. The sample of semen (which is only the carrier for the sperm, and not the sperm itself) is put under a microscope. The laboratory technician then checks the number in eight sample "boxes" under observation. If there are one hundred in these counting chambers, the count represents one hundred million sperm per cubic centimeter, a good high count. If there are only fourteen sperm on view, this is indicative of only fourteen million per cc, not a very good count. A sperm count of 20 million per cc is considered to be the minimum number necessary for good odds that one sperm will survive and fertilize the egg. However, results can vary, and repeated tests over a period of months are often recommended.

But the count isn't everything. The size of the sample—usually ranging from a half to a full teaspoon—is also important, though not as important as the concentration of sperm. Some specimens can be lower than the minimum volume, yet have a high concentration of sperm. Some may have a high volume, but a low concentration. The most important factor is the concentration of the sperm, along with what is called the motility, or the number of units that are active and rapid in movement.

Every sample has a share of sperm that are lifeless and motionless, and some that are misshapen, broken or immature. These cannot make the grade at all, yet are harmless otherwise and present no genetic problem. It is generally believed that you need about 80 percent normal morphology, or active-appearing sperm, and 80 percent motility, sperm moving in a good forward motion.

While I waited for the report on John's test, the only negative thought that kept popping into my mind was how I would *ever* get John back for a second or third count, if they were needed. At my last visit, the doctor had reminded me once again how males feel extremely threatened by workups. He went on to explain how husbands of his patients are often responsible for a good share of the problems. It seems that after they've been trying for a while with no results and the days of maximum fertility, when intercourse is a must, roll around, the husbands often become uptight or, in his words, impotent.

So far I had been lucky. John didn't know anything about the circles we had been stacking up on my maximum fertility days. On days 11, 13, 15, and 17 I would just sidle up and he was none the wiser. But now that John knew about the temperature charts and circles, I would no longer be able to do that. I had no idea how this would psychologically affect John the next time we were up for a circle.

And that next time was coming up. My doctor said that as soon as we got John's test result I was to phone him, report his count per milliliter, and then he would set up my next appointment for step number two in the workup. It was called a postcoital.

This test is performed around the time of ovulation. The couple has intercourse and several hours later the woman is examined by her gynecologist. The procedure is quick, simple, and painless. During a postcoital exam the doctor takes a sample of cervical mucous and examines it under a microscope. What the doctor looks for is the amount of sperm and how they are moving. A good postcoital would reveal the cervical mucous to be thin, clear, watery, and very stretchable, with an abundance of sperm penetrating it. A bad postcoital would show the cervical mucous to be thick and impassable, not allowing the sperm to get through. Or possibly the cervical mucous is good, but there are few sperm or maybe even no sperm. This could indicate an infection, or possibly an allergic reaction.

This was one test I was not looking forward to. One woman I talked to in the doctor's office told me about a friend of hers who made the mistake of telling her husband about the postcoital. It took twenty-seven months of deep analysis to get him stabilized. I planned on telling John about this test. I was sure he could handle it.

Two days later John's doctor phoned with his test result. It was better than good. The doctor told John that he had a sperm count of 70 million per cubic centimeter with 75 percent motility (75 percent were moving in a forward motion) and 80 percent morphology (80 percent of the sperm had a normal oval shape).

This news meant several things. First of all, it meant that John was apparently not responsible for our infertility. Second, I would not have to drag him in for more tests. And third, and most important, his male ego would not be compromised. In fact, after he learned of his test result, I detected an attitude of insufferable pride.

I told Patsy the good news the following day in art class. In between setting up easels and mixing oils she asked, "So how's progress?"

"Patsy, you'll never believe this. John went for the fertility test."

"I bet the poor man wasn't too enthusiastic," she said.

I told her that at first he wasn't, but that after I

explained how important it was he was more or less re-signed to go ahead with it. Then I went on to tell her about the next step, the postcoital, and that at first I wasn't going to tell John about it, but I had given it some thought and had changed my mind. I could no longer do slippery things and, besides, John wasn't like most males. He would surely understand that it just had to be done.

The entire time I had been telling this to Patsy she had been twisting her mouth in an annoying way. I was all set to ask her what the problem was when she plunked down her paint brush, wiped her hands clean with tur-pentine, and spoke.

"Listen Liz, I'm going to skip the fact that in most cases you use good common sense, that you're an intel-ligent woman married to an equally—"

I told Patsy to get to the point.

"What I mean," she said, "is that John might be capable of great understanding. But I'm telling you now, he will harbor deep resentment if he is forced into a sudden sexual situation. In plain and simple words— John must not be told anything about this next test."

In the end, I decided that she might just have a point. But it wasn't *just* because of Patsy's warning that I decided not to tell John about the postcoital. It was also because of that woman in the doctor's office who had told me about her friend's husband and the twenty-seven months of deep analysis it took to get him stabi-lized.

The Postcoital and Other Basic Tests

On the morning of the postcoital test, I ran into an unforeseen complication. Even though I had everything carefully orchestrated for the eight o'clock show, something beyond my control came up. There was no problem with John being too sleepy. He was always up at 4:30. By eight he could usually be heard singing in the kitchen as he scrounged around for his second breakfast.

That morning I needed no alarm clock. I woke at seven, showered, and slipped into something silky. Then at 7:30 I went down to the kitchen and brewed a fresh pot of coffee to give him a quick energy lift.

But when I took the coffee tray up to his office he didn't even look up from his typewriter. He just nodded his head and motioned with one hand for me to drop the tray on the floor. I kicked a few books and papers out of the way to clear space for the tray and left. It was obvious that he was in the middle of a train of thought.

I gave his train of thought ten minutes before I appeared at his door again. It was already 7:50, which meant ten minutes until curtain. This time he looked up and asked, "Are you sick?"

This was not exactly the response I had hoped for.

"No," I said, "do I *look* sick?"

He wanted to know why, if I wasn't sick, I wasn't dressed. Because the clock was running, I began to talk nonsense. I told John how just seeing him at his typewriter made me fall in love with him all over again. Here's where he got suspicious.

"And seeing you in that negligee makes me wonder if it's not a circle morning."

I reassured him that it was definitely *not* a circle day. But now that he mentioned it, it might be a good idea to get a circle—just for the heck of it.

John took a swig of coffee and then looked up out of disbelief. "You mean *you* want to just throw a circle away?" he asked.

"Exactly," I said.

He slipped a piece of manuscript paper in his typewriter and answered, "Good. As soon as I get this last chapter typed and in the eleven o'clock mail."

When I heard eleven o'clock, I could feel my heart sink.

"That means we can't make love until—what time?" I asked.

Now he knew I was up to something. "Eleven," he said. "Maybe eleven-o-five."

"What's the matter with eight? Maybe eight-o-five?"

"Why? Do you have to clear it with the A.M.A.?"

In the end I had to tell him the truth. After a little bit of balking about how it was like making love with an E.K.G. hooked up to his skull, we got our circle. And I was able to get down to my doctor's office by nine.

But once I got down to the office there was another problem. My doctor had been called away on an emergency cesarean. His nurse told me that I could either wait—but it might be quite a long wait—or she could set up another appointment for the following day.

The following day—I couldn't believe that she had actually said that. Didn't she know that a day to the elderly primapara was a lifetime? Didn't she know that I waited for this day the same way a junkie waits for a fix? Didn't she know all the scheming that went into pulling off this stupid test? Didn't she know how paranoid my husband was getting? How paranoid I was getting? How mentally and physically exhausted we were both getting?

I didn't share these thoughts with her. Instead, I just bobbed my head from side to side, as if to say it really didn't matter, but I'd just as soon wait for the doctor anyway. Then I turned away and took a seat along with the others.

I had begun to hate going to that office. I could always count on at least one woman to be wearing one of those maternity T-shirts that says "Baby" with an arrow pointing toward the stomach. As if it weren't bad enough that they came in pregnant, they had to flaunt it too. Those T-shirted women bothered me even more than the ones who came in for their six-week postpartum (after delivery) checkups holding their infants. This made me question whether I wanted to be pregnant more than I actually wanted a baby. Sometimes I had a hard time distinguishing between the two. That wasn't exactly healthy thinking. I often wondered if sick thinking went hand-in-hand with my pregnancy obsession. Maybe I needed a good shrink more than I needed a fertility doctor.

I was just getting ready to fumble around on the table for a magazine when I noticed the same woman I saw the very first time I had come to the office. It was the one I had pegged as a regular, because she was joking with the nurses and calling them by name. Now she was sitting directly across from me. I had wanted to talk to her the last time I had seen her. As I looked up, our eyes met and she smiled. But it wasn't a goony smile— like those of the women who sport those T-shirts. It was a smile of compassion. I knew immediately that she had been this route before.

I have found that the only acceptable reason for

starting up a conversation with a total stranger is for the purpose of griping about something. I can't remember exactly what I began complaining about, but I do remember that I monopolized the entire hour and ten minutes that it took for my doctor to return from his cesarean section. While I was chattering away, I did feel a little badly that I wasn't giving my new friend a chance to share her infertility story too. But I couldn't stop myself. Maybe that's what my friends meant by calling me an unbearable bore. However, this woman didn't appear to be bored. Of course it was the first time she had heard it.

Finally the nurse appeared. My new-found friend was called in first. At least I thought she was my friend. But when she got up from the sofa, I detected a slightly rounded girth underneath a tunic top. This was no friend. She was pregnant. I suddenly felt betrayed. Here I was spilling out intimate details of my workup because I thought that she could identify with me. I had been sure from the way she had been nodding her head that she was one of my kind.

Ever since this obsession had hit me, I had carefully divided the world into two types of people: pregnant and nonpregnant. But then I came to my senses. Perhaps she hadn't told me she was pregnant because she was sensitive to how the nonpregnants felt toward the pregnants. And the only way she could be sensitive was if she had once had a fertility problem herself. But now she was different from me. She belonged to that other half of the world. I hoped that I would never have to run into her again.

All of my anxieties about flunking the postcoital proved to be unfounded. The doctor confirmed that everything *in vivo* appeared to be normal and that we could move on to step number three of the workup.

This time he spared me that plexiglass model of the reproductive system. Instead he used a cardboard diagram that reminded me of a connect-the-dots kids play with. As he followed the dots with his silver pen, he told me that the next test was called a hysterosalpingogram. He threw those seven syllables around three times before he knocked off the medical school jargon and said it was merely an X-ray of the uterus and tubes.

The purpose of the test was to see if my Fallopian tubes were open. He went on to inform me that blocked tubes, frequently the result of an infection, were a major cause of infertility. When he said that, I suddenly recalled a whole section in one of my infertility books devoted to the most common kinds and causes of infection.

Gonorrhea was at the top of the infection list. It is the most destructive of all, simply because it can remain without symptoms and yet insidiously spread throughout the reproductive organs, destroying everything in its path. When this happens it is called Pelvic Inflammatory Disease, or P.I.D. However, if the gonorrhea is caught early, it can be treated with huge doses of penicillin in an effort to protect the tubes. Another type of P.I.D. is caused by bacteria coming from external sources either through an abortion or from the insertion of an I.U.D. Women who wear I.U.D.s have a greater chance of having infections than non-I.U.D. wearers. P.I.D. can also come from internal sources, possibly through a ruptured appendix. Just as in gonorrhea, these other infections may go undetected before the symptoms finally erupt. And when they do, it is often too late. Scarring and adhesions may have already formed on the ovaries and tubes. The only way to safeguard against having an infection turn into P.I.D. is to become aware of the symptoms, such as severe pain in the lower abdomen, and then receive prompt treatment by a gynecologist.

As I was recalling everything I had read about infections, the doctor was describing how the hysterosalpingogram is performed. First a liquid dye that is opaque to X-rays is injected through the cervix, the lower part of the neck of the uterus that protrudes into the vaginal canal. Once the X-ray is taken, the doctor is able to see an outline of the inside of the uterus and the Fallopian tubes. If the tubes are open, the liquid should overflow into the abdominal cavity. He reassured me that this test was only slightly painful and it did not require hospitalization. I was also glad to learn that it did not require John.

I was headed out the office door with my appointment for a hysterosalpingogram when I was suddenly prompted to turn around and ask one last question. I asked the doctor whether the woman who had the appointment right before mine had once been a fertility patient too. As soon as I got those words out, I told him that I realized he couldn't discuss other patients, and I went on to explain my obsession. I told him that ever since I had gotten the urge to have a baby, my rational thinking had taken leave. I was able to think of nothing but getting pregnant. Everything I did now revolved around the days of my maximum fertility. During those four days I was making John's life miserable. In order to be sure that John wouldn't be too tired for a circle, I planned our social life so that we didn't have one. We didn't go out and we didn't have friends over. We were sort of living in the twilight zone of life. The other twenty-four days my life was governed by the basal thermometer. If I had a good temperature reading that indicated a possible pregnancy, I'd have a good day. But if it wasn't a good reading, it would make my life, as well as that of everyone around me, a living hell.

The doctor was very sympathetic. He reassured me that my anxieties were not unique. Infertility is a highly emotional thing for women to go through, and for men too. In fact the emotional problems added another element to the couple's dilemma. He explained that if a woman is overanxious or under extreme stress, this could easily throw off the hypothalamus in the primitive region of the brain and disturb ovulation. I wished he hadn't told me that. Now I had something new to fret over.

From there, he went into the physical problems. He couldn't discuss the patient I had asked about, but he did tell me about a few too many anonymous patients who later went on to become pregnant. I heard about one woman who had blocked tubes. He talked of another's annovulation (the suspension of ovulation) and several cases of endometriosis. To me, however, they were merely textbook case histories.

While he was talking, it suddenly occurred to me that a friend I hadn't seen in over a year had had some sort of fertility problem. In fact, now that I thought about it, I purposely hadn't seen her for that reason—she was always weepy and depressing to be around. Although I couldn't recall whether she had ever gone into any of the details concerning her infertility, I did remember her saying something about a blocked tube. I would give her a call the moment I got home.

Not only did I give Donna a call, but we talked for over an hour. And then we ended the conversation only because we made plans to meet for lunch the following afternoon.

I was so anxious for that lunch that I arrived at the restaurant fifteen minutes too early. But I had things to occupy myself. I always traveled with my temperature charts jammed inside my wallet. While I waited, I reviewed the last three months, trying to pinpoint what could have gone wrong.

Once Donna sat down, we lost no time picking up where our telephone conversation had left off. I couldn't believe that here sat a woman who at one time bored me to death. Now I was hanging on her every word. Everything she said, I felt. We shared a true communion of the souls. Even Patsy, whom I counted on for good, solid, constructive advice, never really understood what I was feeling. But Donna did.

Donna knew what it was like to go through a whole month, scrupulously following all the set procedures to ensure pregnancy, and then on day 28 getting a period. She knew what it was like to be one or two days late, and how you become crazed looking for signs of pregnancy. How you even invent signs that don't exist.

She knew what it was like to be stuck in the same room with a pregnant woman and to have to listen to her belly-ache about her nausea while you sit there and think of how you'd kill for a case of morning sickness. She knew what it was like to *have* to get a circle and for your husband to be out of town, or too tired, or too grouchy, or just too fed up with the whole fertility thing to even want to get a circle.

In fact Donna knew all too well how the workup can affect relationships. Her three year search for fertility left her with neither a baby nor a husband. At thirty-three she was in the process of getting a divorce—a divorce she loosely connected to the keeping of one too many temperature charts.

In between a few tears, Donna told me how she first got the "urge" to have a baby. It was right after her thirtieth birthday. She was home visiting her sister, who had just given birth. Donna recalled looking into the hospital's glass nursery and suddenly feeling as if she were going to cry. This was a feeling she interpreted at the time as one of happiness for her sister—even though she thought her sister was crazy for ever wanting to ruin her life with a baby.

The following day Donna went back to the hospital and peered into the nursery, and the same feeling came over her. This time she realized that her feeling was not so much one of happiness for her sister as it was one of sadness for herself—a sadness that she would never have a baby.

Donna had been married to Bill for seven years. They had both agreed that there were too many kids in the world already, and that their jobs were not conducive to parenting. Donna owned a small boutique and traveled extensively searching for unique objets d'art with which to stock her store. Bill did his share of travel as an advertising manager.

Each month Donna's desire for a baby grew stronger. But because this was so out of character for her, she constantly rationalized it as some sort of temporary mental disorder. It wasn't temporary and it didn't go away. It got worse. Soon she found herself totally fascinated, if not obsessed, with the idea of becoming pregnant. She began studying the pregnant women who came into her store, reading articles on childbirth, and buying books on pregnancy.

Finally she told her husband that she would like to have a baby. After he came out of shock, he agreed, and soon became as enthusiastic as she. But that would not last.

As Donna continued to chronicle her story, I recognized two strong parallels between her situation and mine. First and most obvious was that neither of us had wanted children in our twenties. We had been fulfilled and content without them. And second, the strong "urge" to have them had hit with little warning and no conscious effort when we reached our thirties. This made me more convinced than ever that there really is something to the "maternal instinct."

I was hoping that our parallels would end here. I certainly never wanted to upset my marriage the way Donna had hers. Her husband couldn't handle the fertility workup. I tried to make myself feel better by thinking that, since he was only four years older than Donna, this was because he was still emotionally immature. But then I thought of how John reacted when I told him about the fertility workup.

And John had been a lot luckier than Bill. Bill had to go for three sperm counts before he learned that his count was on the low end of the scale, some 15 million per milliliter against an 80 million average. Donna said that it had been bad enough conning him into going there three times, but when he got his final test score he became indignant and bitter. After Donna saw how he was taking it, she phoned the doctor and pleaded with him to say that there was some sort of a mixup down at the laboratory; that his count was at least average, not scraping the bottom. But the doctor said no. I certainly did not tell Donna about John's better than average count. I felt that that bit of news might ruin the beginning of a good relationship.

During the months of Bill's workup the doctor performed a series of tests to see if he could establish what was causing the low count. The first thing the doctor checked for was a varicocele, which is simply a varicose vein in the scrotum. It is usually located in the left scrotum. This is the single most frequent cause of male infertility, accounting for roughly 40 percent of the problems.

Although there have been no clear-cut theories as to exactly why the swollen vein causes infertility, doctors suspect two reasons. First, the vein causes an elevated temperature in the scrotum, which would affect sperm production. In fact men who don't have a varicocele, but who wear tight underwear or jeans, can also have a low sperm count because their testicles are several degrees too warm for adequate sperm production. When Donna heard that, she immediately replaced all of Bill's jockey shorts with boxer shorts one size too large. She also encouraged him to sit around on a bag of ice while watching TV. Donna had read that that was one way to cool down his private parts.

The second reason doctors think a swollen vein in the testicles may cause infertility is that the blood in the vein flows in the wrong direction. This reverse-action flow causes a metabolic change in the production of sperm. The only way to correct the problem is with surgery. The vein is tied off through a small incision in the groin. The operation is considered to be minor and takes less than half an hour.

After the doctor was certain that Bill did not have a varicocele or any other obstruction, he began treating him with the hormone Clomid, the same drug given to women to stimulate ovulation. In both men and women, the drug helps to activate the hypothalamus and to stimulate the pituitary gland to release two hormones, FSH and LH. In the male, these two hormones stimulate sperm production. However, the Clomid treatment is controversial. It has not been as dramatically successful in increasing sperm counts as it has been in inducing ovulation in women.

In addition to the hormone treatment, Bill's doctor suggested that they abstain from sex until Donna's most fertile days. In other words, to "stockpile," a technique that is also highly controversial, since adequate sperm replacement takes only forty-eight hours.

Bill's doctor also suggested that once his sperm count improved they could further increase their chances at conception by trying artificial insemination by the husband or the AIH (the artificial insemination husband). This was not to be confused with AID, insemination by a donor. But in order for the husband insemination to be effective, the male's sperm count must be strong enough to make conception a possibility.

The AIH procedure is performed in the gynecologist's office right around the time of ovulation. Ovulation is determined in two ways: by keeping the temperature chart, and by the doctor examining the cervical mucous to make sure it is thin and elastic so that the sperm can swim through it. Once the correct time is determined, the doctor takes the husband's sperm and places it on the wife's cervix. The way this is most commonly done is to fit a small plastic cup over the cervix and inject the semen through a long hollow stem attached to the plastic cup. In effect, this doubles the husband's sperm count, since the semen never touches the vagina. Bathing the cervix surrounded by the cup in semen ensures that the majority of the sperm have direct access to the endocervical canal and that they are not killed by the acidity of the vagina. This is usually done two or three times around ovulation.

Donna mentioned that Bill hadn't told her about the artificial insemination his doctor recommended. She had found a typed sheet of paper stuffed into his sport jacket pocket.

Donna said that she hadn't wanted to press her luck, so she mentioned nothing. Besides she was not without her own set of fertility problems. She was on step three of her workup, which featured the hysterosalpingogram, the X-ray of the uterus. Donna was an outpatient in the X-ray department of the hospital when her test was performed. It had been timed to be a week after her period so that the uterine lining would not be too thick. An overly developed lining could hamper the free flow of the dye through the tubes. It would also be done before ovulation so that there would be no chance of conception taking place; the radiation coming from an X-ray could cause possible harm to the developing fetus.

Donna said that she had been so anxious about the test that her period dragged on an extra three days. Her doctor said that that was one of the side effects of infertility testing, but that since her period had stopped they would go ahead and perform the test as scheduled. Her doctor also warned her that the hysterosalpingogram might be somewhat painful, and that she could ask for a local anesthetic of the cervix if she felt she needed it. But once Donna got to the hospital, she decided to skip the local and deal with the pain.

The doctor began the test by taking an X-ray of Donna's abdomen before injecting the dye. This is done to make sure that there is nothing inside her abdominal cavity that could be confused with the dye that would soon be injected through an instrument in her cervix.

Donna said that the test was done under a fluoroscope screen so that, as the dye was being injected, the doctor could see on a TV screen whether it was flowing freely down through the tubes. If it wasn't, this could mean that there was an obstruction in the tubes. A common obstruction would be adhesions, which can usually be corrected through surgery. The doctor also looks for obstructions in the uterus; they too can usually be corrected through surgery. Occasionally the doctor would stop to take an X-ray from various angles in order to have a permanent record.

Donna said that her own doctor had warned her that she might feel some unpleasant uterine cramping as the test was being performed and that these cramps could last for several hours. But the only sensation Donna experienced was a feeling of fullness in her abdomen, as if her period were about to start.

The results of the hysterosalpingogram were normal, which meant it was time to move on to step four of the workup, the laparoscopy. This is a surgical operation in which a thin telescopelike instrument equipped with light and lens is inserted through the naval to examine the tubes and other pelvic organs.

I didn't miss a word as Donna told me about her operation. I suddenly felt like my grandmother. The only time I could ever get her full attention was when I was discussing funerals, terminal illness, or operations of more than eight stitches. But unlike my grandmother, I had a good reason for interest in Donna's laparoscopy. I would soon be a candidate for this operation.

Donna went on to tell me that the operation had shown an envelope of adhesions running between the ovary and the fimbriated end of the tubes, the part the egg enters after coming out of the ovary. And that during the laparoscopy her doctor was able to sever all the adhesions, making a clear pathway from the ovary to the tube.

After Donna's operation she was more fertile than Bill. Her doctor gave her a 90 percent chance of conceiving—even with Bill's less-than-optimum sperm count. Donna decided not to share the news of just how fertile she was. What she did share with Bill was a somewhat gnarled version of the truth to boost his morale. She told him that her doctor said, even with the operation, he was still the more fertile of the two.

As soon as Bill heard that, his vital life signs returned—almost to the point of his becoming swellheaded. But Donna claimed that the lie was all worth it. I knew what she meant.

Donna said that, for nearly a year after her laparoscopy, she and Bill continued the scheduled sex. But toward the end of that year, she noticed that Bill was
planning more and more business trips out of town.
Donna said that she began accusing him of purposely
planning the trips to be away on her maximum fertility
days. In turn, he began accusing her of being a temper-
ature-taking, paranoid bore. And they both began accusing each other for their inability to have a baby.
Nearly three years after they first began the workup, they
filed for divorce.

Across the table from me, Donna was in tears. So
was I. I tried to think of something to say that would
make her feel better. Finally I began telling her a few
of the things Patsy had said. I told her that kids can be
a real drain, always demanding to be chauffeured around
as if they were four-star generals. When they didn't want
to be driven somewhere, it was because they had invited
an army of miniature commandos over to empty the
refrigerator. I ended by telling Donna that our infertility
was probably a blessing in disguise, and that we should
be celebrating. So we wound up the lunch with another
glass of wine and vowed to meet the following week.

Donna and I not only had lunch that following
week, but every week thereafter for the next three
months. Patsy said that it was a real phenomenon that
we never got bored with one another. She was referring
to the one time I invited her to come along to meet
Donna. Before the coffee was even served, Patsy made
some excuse that she had to get home and fold laundry.

My relationship with Donna came to a temporary standstill. Patsy speculated that it was probably just a case of sensory overload and that I shouldn't worry about it. But I did. I knew what was bothering Donna. The last time we had lunch, she mentioned that she had been giving some thought to having a baby with or without a husband. At the time she said that, I didn't think that she was really serious. I laughed it off with some comment on our mutual Catholic school upbringing. I asked her what she thought the Little Sisters of the Inquisition would say if they could hear her now. Then to make things worse I went on to question her on exactly what she intended to tell her future child about his or her father. By the time I realized just how sensitive she was on the point, the damage had been done.

I tried during several telephone conversations to make up for my insensitivity by telling her that if I were in her shoes, I'd do the same. And I guess I would have. But I got the distinct feeling from the chill on the other end of the line that Donna didn't believe I really approved. Soon our conversations became fewer and fewer until one day they finally stopped. But that wasn't the end of Donna. She would surface once again in the most unusual way.

4

The Laparoscopy

It wasn't because of anything Donna had said that I decided to skip step three of my workup. If anything, Donna helped allay any fears I might have had. It was simply because I couldn't stand the suspense of step four, the laparoscopy, hanging over my head, or, worse yet, the extra month or maybe two that it would take. From everything I had read, the laparoscopy does basically everything the hysterosalpingogram does and then some. I discussed this with my doctor and he explained that the step-by-step workup was designed to diagnose fertility problems the simplest way first, beginning with the temperature charts and working up to surgery. However, he was sympathetic to my anxieties of wanting to get through the workup as quickly as possible. He said that the hysterosalpingogram was the least important of any of the steps. If I had to skip any, that would be the one. But he did warn that there was still a chance that after the laparoscopy we would have to do a hysterosalpingogram. I told him that I would take that chance.

I didn't even try to explain how emotionally drained I was, to say nothing of the toll this whole thing was taking on John. As it was, whenever he even suspected it was circle time, he would come down with some sort of psychosomatic illness. Just days earlier I had promised John with my life that I no longer kept temperature charts. I didn't like to lie, but in order to preserve his sanity I had to. It had been only a few days after I had reassured him that I was finished with the charts that I had accidentally left them lying on the coffee table where he immediately spotted them.

"So we *are* still keeping copious records, are we?" he said as he waved the dog-eared pieces of paper in the air. I detected more than a bit of cynicism in his voice.

"More or less." I tried grabbing them. But it was too late. He had a vise grip on them. I was now just praying that he wouldn't notice the notes I had scribbled at the bottom of each sheet.

"That damn doctor of yours is still looking over my shoulder."

"It's important." Again I tried reaching for the charts. Again he tightened his grip.

"You're not taking these charts in looking like this, are you?"

John was referring to the fact that there weren't enough circles. I tried pointing out to him that that was because we had to save up the first eleven days. Then when two of our four circle days rolled around, he had been too tired meeting his writing deadline to meet our circle deadline. And then from days sixteen onward, *I* had been too emotionally sapped to even think about a circle.

I was sure that he understood. But I was wrong.

"Okay," he said, "you can have the charts back if you fill in a few more circles."

"No deal."

"We'll make up for it another time."

"That's cheating."

I began making a joke out of the whole thing by pointing out to him how ridiculous it was. He began to see the humor, that is, until he noticed the chicken scratch at the bottom of the page.

"What's this?" he asked.

"What's what?"

Then he began to decipher my notes. They read:

Day 11. John came to bed. Very tired. Tried but no luck. Day 12. Good night rest. Got circle. Day 13. John had slight cold and temperature. No circle. Day 14. John ached all over but got circle . . .

"Obsession, thy name is woman," he said. And he dropped the charts and went upstairs to his office.

That was the last thing I heard him say for the rest of the afternoon. I wished he had screamed and carried on. His silence was always a killer. I followed him upstairs explaining how those notes were just like the footnotes he puts at the bottom of his manuscripts. And that they were just my own personal reminders of how things went. But the more I said, the quieter he became.

By that evening the silence broke. I'm not so sure that was any better. He started off by offering to buy me a microscope and two fruit flies so that I wouldn't be bored between circle days. Then he went on to say that when friends stopped him in the street to ask "how's it going," he could just show them the charts. He even accused me of showing Patsy the charts. And that I denied with my life. Another small lie.

John's anger did not last. But his paranoia did. I was just glad that the circle days for that month were over, and that there would be no circle days the following month, because I was going into the hospital for my laparoscopy.

The next two weeks were difficult. John became suspicious of my every move. He began reading slippery things into my innocent actions. Fortunately I had Patsy to go to for some good sound advice.

First of all, she couldn't believe that I had left the charts lying around for John to find. Then she said that she bloody well understood how poor John was being affected. But since the damage had been done, I should stop dwelling on it. And for heaven's sake, I should quit

running around the house after him explaining that I
just kept notes because it was the most important thing
in my life. She warned me that that alone would finish
him off.

Although Patsy sympathized with John, she also
understood my obsessional behavior. She told me how
she had been almost as obsessional over *not* getting
pregnant.

After Patsy was certain I had taken all of her advice
in, she mumbled something about having to hurry and
get home. Her two sons would be waiting to be chauffeured to town. Then she had to pick up her daughter
and friends and drive them back from town. Her parting
words were to the effect that kids can't stand to see a car
sitting in the garage with its tires cooling down, and that
my turn was coming up.

I wasn't so sure that my turn at having a baby was
coming up, but it was my turn to go into the hospital
for the laparoscopy. This surgery is euphemistically
called a "Band-Aid" operation, an annoying name for
surgery even though the incision is actually small enough
to be covered with a single Band-Aid. I didn't mind the
actual surgery as much as the thought of going under a
general anesthetic. My doctor reassured me that with
today's modern anesthetic techniques the risk was very
small. He said that it was common for his patients to be
apprehensive about the process, and that some women
had even cancelled three times. But later they all went
on to have successful laparoscopies that enabled them

to become pregnant. Knowing that others had experienced the same fears and had come out of it with babies was the only thing that lessened my own anxieties.

The morning of my laparoscopy my mother phoned to tell me that she had been praying for me and that the night before she dreamt I would have a baby.

I had put off telling my mother about the fertility problem for several months. I was afraid that she would say something like, "What do you expect when you wait till middle age to have a baby?" Or she may have just felt sorry for me. That would have been worse.

Instead, she told me her own story of infertility, a story I was hearing for the very first time.

My parents were married for four years before my older brother came along. Every month for those four years, my parents tried to conceive, but without luck. My mother recalled that thirty-five years ago you didn't discuss your fertility problems, especially if you were Irish Catholic. In those days if you didn't have a baby the problem was exclusively the woman's. The only thing my mother's gynecologist told her was to relax and she would get pregnant. He never even suggested that my father see a urologist; this probably had something to do with male bonding. He didn't want to inflict that kind of torture on one of his own kind.

The only person my mother felt she could confide in was my father's mother. She went on to tell me that on the first Friday of every month my grandmother and she would go to St. Ann's for mass. After the service, my grandmother would double bless herself with Holy

Water, genuflect, then drop by the statue of the Blessed Virgin, the patron saint of motherhood. Clutching a pair of white pearl rosary beads, she would pray for my mother to have a baby.

After my grandmother was certain that the Blessed Virgin had heard her, she would nudge my mother to let her know that it was time to light the candles. Once in front of the rows of small candles, my grandmother would reach into her black coin purse, daintily pinch out a dime, and drop it into the tin box. Then she would light two candles—even though a dime only bought you one candle. One candle was for my mother and one was for her baby.

This ritual continued for nearly three years. Then one day my mother found out she was pregnant. Since my father was at work, the first person to hear was my grandmother. That afternoon, they celebrated at St. Ann's. Once inside the church my grandmother was so excited that she rushed directly to the candles without even a pit stop at the Blessed Virgin.

My grandmother lit the two candles, quickly genuflected, and was ready to leave so that she could spread the word, without dropping in the dime. My grandmother explained that she had been dimeing it for four years and that the Blessed Virgin knows better than anyone how expensive it is to raise a child, and that it was now time to start saving the dimes. Then she pushed a dime inside my mother's hands and closed her fingers over it.

As John drove me to the hospital for the laparoscopy, I thought about that dime story and how simple life must have been thirty-five years ago: you merely prayed to the Blessed Virgin, and the rabbit died.

As we turned onto the tree-lined parkway, I thought of how much better things were today, at least from a medical standpoint. My mother hadn't been given the chance to have a workup. In fact she never even dreamed that there was such a thing.

While John was listening to the morning news on the car radio, grimacing at the fighting going on in the Middle East, I felt ashamed that I really couldn't feel anything for anyone else's problems, regardless of how monumental. This baby craving was dwarfing everything around me. I thought about how, at one time, I would have been happy to adopt. But in the state I was in, if someone offered me a newborn infant, I think I would have turned it down for the chance of having my own. That's what bothered me. I was still confused as to whether I wanted to be a mother or I just wanted to be pregnant and give birth.

Thirty minutes after we left our house, we swung into the hospital's emergency entrance. John dropped me off, and then went to park the car. I waited next to the receptionist's long white desk, just inside the sliding glass doors. To kill time, I began eavesdropping on a policeman who was telling two nurses about his recent trip to Las Vegas.

For the first time that morning, my mind turned away from myself. But that didn't last. The minute I spotted John coming in from the parking lot, my mind went right back to the laparoscopy. I was worried that the whole bothersome operation might not show clearly if anything was wrong. I was counting on the doctor finding something wrong so that there would be something specific to correct. There was always the threat that I might be one of that small percentage for whose unfertility the doctor had no explanation. I had recently read that when doctors can't find out what is wrong, it doesn't mean that there isn't anything wrong. It simply means that medical science has not advanced far enough to detect the problem.

We wound our way around several sterile green corridors before we arrived at my room, which was in the old section of the hospital. Before I even had a chance to break out into a cold sweat, a nurse entered and handed me a white gown. She instructed me to take off everything and then get into bed. The anesthesiologist would be in shortly to take my medical history, and then my own doctor to brief me on the surgery. While I was getting into the gown, John was turning the room upside down looking for an ashtray. He ended up using his hand.

Moments after the anesthesiologist left, the nurse came back clutching a miniature paper cup that contained a pill that was supposed to make me relax. It worked. By the time my doctor showed up I was so relaxed that I wasn't even nervous about what John was going to say to him. It was the first time John and the fertility doctor were meeting. When the doctor shook hands with John and asked him how he was doing, John started to say not bad. But then he hesitated and said that he'd have to check the charts and circles again. Fortunately they both laughed.

After a bit of small talk, consisting mainly of the doctor reassuring John that he knew of no fertility patient's husband who had ended up with permanent psychological damage, he began to explain what the operation would involve.

First a dose of short-term anesthetic is administered. Then the doctor exposes the cervix, opening it just enough to get a sample of the lining of the uterus for study by the pathologist in order to diagnose for endometriosis. Since the hysterosalpingogram had not been done, the inside of the uterus would be examined to make sure there is no obstruction. Then a hairline incision a half-inch long is made in the depths of the navel. A long hollow needle is then passed into the perinatal cavity. Following that, carbon dioxide is blown through the needle, inflating the abdomen, creating room to give a clearer picture of the pelvic organs. After that, a long telescopelike instrument equipped with light and lens is inserted through that same incision. This instrument illuminates the abdominal cavity, providing a bird's eye view of the whole pelvic area.

The doctor went on carefully outlining each step of the laparoscopy. He told me that he would be looking at the size, shape, and contour of all the pelvic organs, checking carefully for patches of endometriosis on the bladder, tubes, ovaries, and the lining of the abdominal cavity, especially behind the uterus. Since the endometrium normally lines the uterus he would be looking for it only in abnormal places, such as the tubes, ovaries, and abdomen. In addition to the endometriosis factor, he would be looking for adhesions and scarring on the uterus and Fallopian tubes and ovaries, other major causes of infertility. And just as in the hysterosalpingogram, dye would be injected through the cervix to rule out tubal blockage.

He went on to explain that the reason he had scheduled the operation precisely for the eighteenth day of my cycle was so he could also see if there was a recently formed corpus luteum covering the ovaries. The corpus luteum is a yellow mass that forms on the surface of the ovaries following ovulation. It is this yellow mass that is responsible for the production of the hormone progesterone during the second half of the monthly cycle. The corpus luteum is necessary to prepare the uterine lining for the implantation of the fertilized egg. Without it, implantation cannot take place.

I had never anticipated that getting pregnant could be so complicated, especially in light of the sex-education classes we were given in Catholic school. As I look back, if the Virgin birth were a hard one to swallow, it was nothing compared to Sister Mary Agnes's trumped-up version of how babies were conceived.

She claimed that when God decided it was time for you to have a baby, He asked Mary if she thought you would raise your child in the One, Holy, Catholic and Apostolic Church.

Sister Mary Agnes went on to say that after Mary had kept tight surveilliance on you, she would report back to God. If God was satisfied, He would tell Mary to pick a saint who would sprinkle a seed on you as you slept. Sister Mary Agnes thought that the saint would probably arrive through the window around two in the morning, when all the lights were off. And nine months later you would have a baby.

You would then name your baby after the saint who sprinkled you. Sister Mary Agnes left a lot of holes in her story. For years after I was scared to sleep with the lights off for fear some joker saint would accidentally come through my window sprinkling the fairy dust.

Before the doctor left to scrub, he asked if we had any questions. I didn't, but John did. He wanted to know what my chances were of becoming pregnant. The doctor depersonalized his answer. He told us that, according to recent statistics, over 60 percent of the couples who are treated conceive, and that this percentage is on the rise.

Soon after the doctor left, two nurses came in. This time I got a shot to relax me even further and one of those paper hats you tuck all your hair under. In a drifting euphoria, I was wheeled down the corridor to the elevator that would take me to the operating room. John was at my side telling me what a brave person I was. He looked as if *he* were the one going under the knife. Finally we got to the elevator. Just as it opened, John leaned over, gently kissed my forehead, and told me that he would be back at the room praying for me to have that baby.

Once out of the elevator, I was pushed down another long corridor and then through a set of electronically controlled double doors before arriving at a holding area just outside the operating room. I was in that area only a matter of minutes when I saw a green scrub suit approaching and I recognized my doctor's voice. Before I had a chance to tell him that I was suddenly frightened all over again about receiving the anesthetic, he held my hand and began telling me a joke I had heard several times before. Out of nervousness I started laughing. I felt as if my knees were shaking in time with the laughter. Before he got to the punch line, a young male attendant appeared and wheeled me feet first into the operating room. It was a spacious white-tiled room with a huge light hanging over the operating table and shiny metal equipment scattered on equally shiny tables.

My stretcher pulled up beside the operating table. I was told to slide onto it. There were three or four others in surgical gowns and masks in the room. While they were doing something with various instruments, they were casually discussing where to get the best Chinese food in town. I couldn't believe that they were talking about anything so frivolous in the operating room, but then again they weren't getting operated on. Suddenly the doctor was at my side again. I was all set to ask him if he was sure I would wake up again, but instead I asked him the punch line of his joke.

Within minutes the anesthesiologist arrived. He told me that I would feel a slight prick in my left arm where the I.V. would go in. After they taped it down, several little plastic suctions were taped onto my chest to monitor my heartbeat. Then my blood pressure was checked. Finally the anesthesiologist, who was at my left side, said that I was going to go to sleep. The last thing I remember was a very funny taste in my mouth.

CHAPTER 5

Fertility Drugs

The next thing I remembered was waking up in the recovery room with a nurse squashed between some sort of monitor and my bed, poking at my fingernails. Because I was still a little doped up, I thought she was looking at my ragged manicure. I jerked my hand away and explained that I typed a lot. It wasn't until later that I realized she was just checking to see if my vital life signs were returning.

As soon as my eyes focused, I noticed my doctor off in the corner of the room. He was sitting at a desk writing furiously. I must have called over to him a little too loudly, because the nurse taking my pulse jumped.

He called back to the nurse, asking if Elizabeth was still yakking away. Then he came over and asked what I meant by "a dime and a saint." I must have been trying to tell them about my mother's fertility story and how she and my grandmother had prayed for a baby. I had told them just about half the story when I fell back asleep.

I didn't learn the results of my laparoscopy until several hours later when my doctor phoned my room from his office. All the pelvic organs appeared to be normal in size, shape, and contour. There was no trace of endometriosis, scarring, or adhesions on the uterus or Fallopian tubes. The dye flowed freely through both tubes, indicating that they were functioning normally. That was the good news.

The bad news—which was really good news—was that he had found the problem. He could not see a hole in the corpus luteum from which an egg had been released. I was making hormones, which was indicated by the rise in my temperature charts, but the mechanical release of the egg was being interfered with for some unknown reason. In other words, I was having a faulty ovulation.

In order for ovulation to occur, several things have to happen. First, the hypothalamus in the brain must activate the pituitary gland (a gland located at the base of the brain). Once the pituitary is activated, it in turn produces two of the hormones necessary for a normal cycle, FSH and LH. They are responsible for stimulating the egg inside the ovary to ripen, mature, and then emerge from the surface of the ovary. After the egg leaves the ovary, the ovary becomes covered with the yellow mass, corpus luteum.

While my doctor continued his vivid description of the intricate reproductive process, I began to wonder how anyone ever got pregnant. Just one hormone could be slightly out of kilter, and ovulation would be thrown off. This made me contemplate the miracle of birth. It also made me contemplate all those recent TV specials devoted to the epidemic of teenage pregnancies. The interviews are always the same. They depict several pregnant teenage girls, in profile so as to not reveal their identities. The girls unanimously agree on one thing: they are shocked to learn that they could actually get pregnant the first time they "did it."

This epidemic made me question more than ever whether my infertility was directly related to my age. The *New York Times* ran a study by French physicians that indicated that 73 percent of women who were twenty-five and under have successful conceptions. But the group I belonged to, including those between thirty-one and thirty-five, have only a 61 percent success rate. And worse yet, the group I was soon to join, the elderly primapara's of thirty-five and older, had only a 53 percent rate of success.

I was waiting for my doctor to wrap up his lengthy essay on reproduction. I wanted to ask him why I wasn't releasing any eggs. Was it because of my age? Or had I always had the problem? But before I had a chance to ask him those questions, he told me he was going to prescribe a fertility drug that would start ovulation. It was called clomiphene citrate (Clomid). When he said fertility drug, I thought "litter." Then I thought it was a stroke of luck that John had stepped out of the room for a cigarette. John had come a long way. Just hours earlier when I was being carted off to the operating room, he had shocked me by saying that he would be back at the room praying for me to have a baby. Whether or not he really meant it, I will never know. But I do know that he would never say that he was going to pray for me to have more than one baby. This set up quite a conflict within me.

But the conflict was short-lived. According to my doctor, Clomid was very mild. At best, it would produce twins. It was not like the powerful fertility drug Pergonal, which was responsible for all the quadruplets and quintuplets I had read about in the supermarket checkout lines. Later I read that Pergonal was first isolated in a convent by an Italian chemist. He used the urine of old Roman nuns to extract a substance known as HMG (human menopausal gonadrotropin). HMG is capable of bypassing the pituitary and directly stimulating the ovaries to release multiple eggs. This is the reason for quintuplets. I was wondering what the reason was for using the nuns. A convent seems an awfully strange place for developing a fertility drug.

Clomid was one of the biggest breakthroughs in infertility, causing 70 to 80 percent of the women treated to ovulate. It is used to solve a variety of problems, including annovulation (the absence of ovulation) and progesterone deficiencies, as well as to control the time of ovulation.

How Clomid works is quite simple. The synthetic hormone activates the pituitary gland to release increased amounts of FSH and LH. These two hormones in turn stimulate the ovaries to release an egg. The drug merely gives nature a nudge.

John and I left the hospital at five o'clock, only ten hours after I had first arrived. Although some laparoscopy patients stay overnight, my doctor felt that since he didn't have to perform any additional surgery, I could go home that same afternoon.

When I stood up to put on my jeans, I felt a tinge of nausea left over from the anesthetic and some tenderness around the middle. But any really uncomfortable sensations were overshadowed by my optimism that pregnancy was only a few Clomid treatments away. I would begin the Clomid in six weeks, taking a total of five pills each month. The first tablet would be taken on day five of the cycle, and the remaining pills on the four consecutive days thereafter.

During the following six weeks, my life reverted to what it had been like before the workup. John was showing fewer signs of paranoia, and I was less obsessive. There was a reason for this more relaxed atmosphere. During the six weeks between the laparoscopy and the start of the Clomid, I had been liberated from the temperature charts, basal thermometer, and the scheduled circle days. For the first time in almost two years I saw real hope for getting pregnant.

Only one thing troubled me. I hadn't been the first to tell John about the Clomid. The day I was supposed to pick up my prescription, the druggist phoned to say he didn't have any more tablets in stock and could I come by the following morning. Unfortunately, I hadn't been home to get that message; but John was.

When I returned home, it took me half the evening to calm him down enough so that I could explain that Clomid was not like the powerful fertility drugs he had read about. The most we could have on Clomid were twins, and there was less than a 10 percent chance of that.

Three months after I started using Clomid, there were still no signs of pregnancy. But I wasn't discouraged. My doctor had warned me when I first went on the Clomid not to expect instant success. It often takes many months to achieve a regular ovulatory cycle.

But then in the fourth month something happened. My period was late. I was sure this meant I had conceived. The Clomid must have worked, and fortunately so had John. We had gotten our three circles at just the perfect time. Everything was ideal for a pregnancy.

I phoned my doctor with the good news. Although he was pleased, he cautioned that I was only *one* day late and I shouldn't get overly excited. He said I should wait a week and if I still hadn't gotten my period I should come in for a blood test. Regardless of his warning, I got excited. The following three days were the longest in my life. I became conscious of every muscle twinge. I woke up with telltale signs of morning sickness and went to bed craving weird foods. John swore I even began walking like a ninth-month pregnant woman. I must have phoned Patsy every hour to ask her if she could try to remember how she felt at the very beginning of her pregnancies. But she was no help. All she said was "first panic, then depression." The last time I phoned I asked her if nausea comes in the first couple weeks of pregnancy. She didn't answer me. Instead, she went on to say that she had just returned from the A&P where she had been standing at the check-out line behind a woman she described as a "vision." She had on a Perry Ellis sweater, a Norma Kamali skirt, and Joan-and-David pumps.

It always amazed me the way Patsy could spot designer clothes. She continued to say that there she was in her Army-Navy jeans and her son's down jacket. Her grocery cart was overflowing with sugary breakfast cereals, economy-size rolls of toilet tissue, and cartons of cola. On the other hand, the "vision" had a civilized amount of groceries. And certainly nothing that could endow the test-tube rat with hyperglycemia. I told Patsy that that was interesting but I didn't see how it connected.

She said that it connected quite simply. The woman in the Perry Ellis sweater had it all together. She obviously had a good job to support her good taste. Patsy said that she knew she had no children because any woman with kids would not be allowed through the front door without Twinkies and white rubber bread. That woman didn't wake up in the morning, look into the mirror and see that she had let valuable years slip by, with nothing accomplished. She was out there *doing* it.

I felt Patsy was just saying all those things to make me feel better—just in case I wasn't pregnant. Patsy never told me the positive points. She didn't have to. I saw it. I watched her play touch football on their front lawn in the summer. I saw her sled down their driveway with the kids in the winter. And I saw the look in her eyes when her youngest boy came home from school and handed her a bunch of wild flowers that he had picked along the way.

When my period was four days late, I again phoned the doctor's office. I told the nurse that this could mean only one thing: I was pregnant. But she wasn't quite as optimistic. She tried to discourage my coming in for a pregnancy test, saying that I should really try to give it another few days just in case the cycle was running amok. I told her I couldn't wait that long. I was already driving my husband and friends crazy, to say nothing of the mental torture I was putting myself through. As long as a blood test could detect pregnancy ten days after conception, I wanted to end the suspense. She reluctantly told me to be at the office by eleven. At five o'clock that afternoon, she phoned with the results. I was not pregnant. The next day I got my period.

When two more months went by, I began to question whether the fertility problem lay with me or with John. I thought back to how Donna had to send Bill for three counts and was going to send him for a fourth, but he refused point blank to go. Even though John's test had been good, I thought that, since almost nine months had elapsed, perhaps something happened to lower the count. I was seriously considering having him checked out again. But first I thought I had better discuss it with Patsy. I don't know why I always went to Patsy before John. At the time it just seemed like the logical thing to do. She was a detached third party who could look at the situation and remain unemotional.

Several days later John and I were at a party given by Arlene, my art teacher. The party was in honor of Patsy's husband, Donal, who had just completed a two-year run as the doctor in the *Elephant Man* and was opening his one-man George Bernard Shaw play that evening. After dinner we would all be going to the opening night.

I certainly hadn't intended to burden Patsy with my problem at her husband's opening performance. I knew that she had been through her share of grief with Donal preparing for his limited engagement. Whenever I complained about how difficult it was to live with a writer, she told me that it couldn't be worse than living with the *Elephant Man's* doctor, who was now metamorphosing into George Bernard Shaw.

If Donal's stentorian actor's voice hadn't been drowning out all sound, I wouldn't have begun talking so connivingly to Patsy. But since we were sitting on the floor together picking at chicken wings I took the opportunity to ask her what she thought about John going for another fertility test. I was in the middle of telling her what his count was when suddenly I looked up and there was John. Apparently he had heard the entire conversation. Without saying a word to us, he walked over to the other side of the room and began chatting with a few friends, all the while glaring at me.

The following day, Patsy told me that a couple of times during the party she had tried starting up a conversation with John, but had gotten nowhere. When she asked him how he's been, he merely said that she ought to know. And when she asked him how his book was going, he told her that he hadn't been able to concentrate for the last nine months. She said that even Donal had mentioned how odd John had acted at the party. Donal had innocently asked him what his new project was, and John had defensively told him to go ask Elizabeth. Patsy went on to warn that I could never get John in for another fertility test, that I should just back off and give him some breathing space. But only weeks after Patsy had given me that advice, things began to change.

6

Miscarriages

I never dreamed that getting pregnant would become such a priority that I would put my life on hold until that time arrived. Before I got involved in the workup, I had given myself a cut-off date when I would give up the idea of having a baby. Instead, I would go on to do something really great with my life. What that would be I had not yet decided. But the cut-off date came and went. I had now extended it another three months.

Just before this self-imposed extension ran out, my hopes rose as my temperature stayed up, indicating that I just might be pregnant. This time I waited longer than four days after missing my period to have the blood test. I waited five. All the signs pointed toward a pregnancy. I had no doubt that *this* time I had conceived. I told that to the nurse when I phoned to make the appointment for the pregnancy test. But she reminded me that I had had all the same symptoms three months earlier. Then she mentioned something about a psychological pregnancy, that it is a recognized medical phenomenon and that she had seen several such cases. It happens in women who are severely frustrated by the inability to conceive. I politely listened as she went on to tell me that these women manifest all the symptoms of a pregnancy, and only a negative blood test will convince them that their subconscious minds are playing tricks on them. After she finished I asked her if she could squeeze me in for a morning blood test. She did.

After the blood test, I decided to stop off at Lord & Taylor to pick up some bath towels. But before I got to the linen department I made a quick stop to check out the fall line in the infant section. I was hoping that I wouldn't run into the saleslady with the red bun. Every time I had seen her, she had quizzed me on whether I was shopping for myself or a friend. At least she didn't say grandchild. Each time I told her I was shopping for myself. And each time she would invariably glance down at my midriff as if to say, "So where's the baby?" Fortunately she wasn't on duty.

I was in the process of looking at the micro-jogging suits. They caught my eye because they were exact replicas of the kind John always wore. I held one up trying to imagine John and the baby in their matching running suits when suddenly my name was shouted.

"Elizabeth!"

I looked up and there was Donna. But it wasn't the Donna I had known. It was a six-month pregnant Donna.

"I can't believe it." I couldn't think of anything else to say.

Donna threw her arms around me. I guessed she had forgiven me for my insensitivity so many months ago. I also guessed from the looks of her that she had meant every word about having a baby with or without a husband.

After she unclutched me, she led me over to the counter where there were stools to sit on. Donna plopped down several tiny garments, handed the gray-haired saleslady her credit card and began telling me what she had been up to for the last nine months. During Donna's chronicle, the grandmotherly saleslady had been standing in front of us, delicately removing the price tags and folding the baby gear neatly into boxes. Every so often she would look up and smile at Donna's enthusiasm. That is until Donna began to touch on how she had made her decision to get pregnant without marrying her new man. At that point the saleslady's lower jaw dropped open like an unlatched breadbox. I thought before the poor woman keeled over I would steer Donna to the coffee shop.

Once we sat down, Donna told me how she had met Larry several months before she and Bill were divorced. Unlike Bill, Larry was not afraid to show emotion. However, Donna did have to admit that a big part of Bill's problem had been caused by the workup. Donna made it clear that Larry had no sexual hangups. Sex had never been better. I told Donna that that was apparent. She looked down at her pregnant stomach and laughed. I liked Donna much better now that she was pregnant. In fact I couldn't recall if I had ever seen nonpregnant Donna smile.

As we drank coffee Donna told me that she and Larry might marry one day. Apparently Larry was married and had two children. He no longer loved his wife, but he didn't hate her either. As soon as his kids were off to college, he planned on divorcing her and marrying Donna. But from what I gathered, his kids were still in elementary school. It didn't seem to bother Donna that Larry and she might never be married.

During the hour I spent with Donna she talked at length about her amniocentesis test, the procedure to screen for genetic defects, which occur more often in women over thirty-four. She talked about the prepared-childbirth course she had registered to take during her last two months. And she even told me that she had decided against having Larry come into the delivery room. Giving birth would be more of a communion between her and her baby.

For the first time, I realized that her baby was her real love. Donna had simply done the most natural and honest thing in the world. She was not going to be denied the chance to have a baby just because she happened to be single.

At last Donna asked how things were going between John and me. I began by telling her how unfairly I had been treating John over the previous few months. And I seemed to get progressively worse as my desire for a baby grew. Each time I got my period, I would take my disappointment out on him. One month he brought me home a single rose. I accused him of treating my grief lightly. The next month he didn't react. I accused him of being indifferent. I was at my worst around the days of maximum fertility. It was the only time of the month where I felt as if I had any control over the situation.

I went on to tell Donna that on one circle day, I got into bed with knee socks and a terry cloth robe. John took one look at me and said that he felt as if he were in the ring with a frazzled lightweight prizefighter. I began crying and accused him of trying to duck out of the most important circle night of the month. I hated this schizoid behavior, but I couldn't seem to change. I felt trapped with no way out, except of course to have a baby.

I continued to tell Donna that for a third of each month I would become gripped with a fear that I might never have a baby. I might have to live out my life deprived of the one thing I had promised myself when I was given my Tiny Tears doll: a real baby. All the while Donna just kept nodding her head, as if to say she knew exactly what I was talking about.

Finally I told her that perhaps if I hadn't been showered with dolls, doll carriages, doll houses, and doll clothes I wouldn't have had this obsession to be a mother. Donna said that maybe if we had been given erector sets instead of dolls, we would have become iron workers somewhere outside Pittsburgh.

The only thing I didn't tell Donna was that I had just come from having a pregnancy blood test. The last time I had the test, I phoned about ten people and later had to phone them all back with the bad news. This time I wasn't going to make the same mistake.

As I drove home from Lord & Taylor, I thought it was a good thing I had bumped into Donna. Not only had it helped renew our friendship, but the time I had spent with her had also helped take my mind off what the results of my blood test would be. The nurse had promised that she would call promptly at five. And at five o'clock the phone rang.

"Elizabeth?" the nurse said. "Are you standing or sitting?"

"I am."

Then the nurse blurted it out.

"Your blood test is positive."

I suddenly couldn't remember if positive meant yes, I was pregnant, or no, I wasn't.

"Positive of what?" I asked.

That's when she confirmed about five times that I was pregnant and that the blood test was 99 percent accurate.

John was taking the 5:05 train back from the city when the news arrived. It was 6:30 before his car pulled into the driveway. I couldn't wait for him to come through the door, so I ran out and shouted to John and the world that I was pregnant. In fact I shouted so loudly that the elderly gentleman who lives across the road poked his head out the front door to see what all the commotion was about. I had always felt that he and his wife wondered what we did in our converted gardener's cottage all day. Now they knew.

The moment John got out of the car he put his arm around my shoulder, kissed the top of my head, and told me that he had just read that the cost of a college education for the year 2000 A.D. would be at least $90,000, and that the kid better be scholarship material.

That night John took a yardstick upstairs to where we intended to have a nursery and measured where the best place for the crib would be. He even pointed out where the safety gates would go and how we would eventually have to put chicken wire on our open decks.

The one thing John refused to do was to look in the book with the color photos and illustrations of what the baby looks like at less than three weeks of age. In fact there is no resemblance to a baby at all; it looks like a three-layered disk, similar to the tiny blobs I used to see on the beach at low tide. The total length is less than an eighth of an inch.

Four weeks later, I visited the doctor's office. This time I wasn't there as an infertility patient. I was there for my first prenatal exam. I no longer sat in corners. I confidently took a seat smack in the center of the room. After I glanced around the office, wondering who the unfortunates were who were there for the workup, I picked up a copy of *Baby Talk* and began to read. I hated myself for being so smug. But somehow I felt I deserved to be.

My doctor informed me that everything appeared normal for the eighth week of pregnancy. It had only been six weeks since conception, but doctors always count from the last missed period. Then he told me that on my next visit he would set up a special machine to detect the fetus's heartbeat. Until that time he strongly suggested that I keep the news of my pregnancy low key. He went on to say that although I shouldn't dwell on this, there is a 10 percent chance that any woman might spontaneously abort (a medical term for miscarriage that occurs before twenty-four weeks of pregnancy). And my chances were double that because I had conceived on Clomid. After the nurse drew some blood, checking to make sure I had no hormonal deficiencies, she set up an appointment for three weeks later.

But I never made my next prenatal visit. On the morning of the tenth week, I woke up with slight nausea. I chalked it up to morning sickness. But by early afternoon I was still nauseated, plus I noticed there was slight bleeding. I didn't panic. I had read about implantation bleeding. This happens when the embryo is attaching itself to the wall of the uterus; in doing so it can break blood vessels, causing a small amount of bleeding. As a precaution I phoned my doctor's office and reported this to the nurse. She told me that I shouldn't be concerned. Many women have some bleeding in early pregnancy. However she did say that if bleeding continued and cramping started, I should come down to the office. I hung up feeling reassured.

The feeling of reassurance didn't last. Shortly after I got into bed the cramping started. At first it was mild. Within a half hour the cramps intensified to the point where I felt as if I were in labor. I put off calling my doctor. Instead I lay in bed feeling as if my whole world was coming down around me. John must have suspected something. He came over to the bedroom from his office, saw the tears, and knew instantly what had happened. He sat down on the bed and held me. There was nothing to say. Later that afternoon he drove me to the doctor's. My pregnancy had ended only ten weeks after it had begun.

During the three months following the miscarriage I became obsessive about reading every book I could find on miscarriages, trying to pinpoint exactly what had happened and how I could prevent the same thing from happening again. But after all my research I finally came to believe that it was just nature's way of preventing an abnormal fetus from being born. And just because I miscarried once didn't mean that I couldn't go on to have a normal, healthy baby the second time. The only thing that bothered me was the fact that women in their thirties tend to have slightly more miscarriages.

For three solid months, Patsy and John had been supportive, sympathetic, and extremely understanding. But then on the fourth month they turned on me because I was becoming more obsessed. They said that enough was enough. I should no longer entertain myself by reading depressing facts on miscarriages. It was time to get on with it. I reluctantly took their advice. The following day, I packed up all my overdue books, hauled them back to the library and paid a huge fine. Somehow I even enjoyed paying the fine. It sort of marked the last time I would be feeling sorry for myself.

At least I thought it was the last time I would be feeling sorry for myself. But six months later a complete rerun of the first miscarriage occurred. The only difference was that the second pregnancy lasted only eight weeks, not ten. I went into another depression, and I had no idea how I would ever climb out.

Fetal Heartbeat

Several weeks after that second miscarriage, Donna phoned. I hadn't seen her since we had run into each other at Lord & Taylor, although I had phoned to tell her that I was pregnant. It seemed as if our pregnancies weren't nearly as binding for a friendship as the camaraderie we shared while going through the workup.

But now, nearly seven months later, Donna phoned to say that she had given birth to a gorgeous seven-pound, ten-ounce baby girl. She had named her Sarah, after her mother. Donna said that she had to do something to make her mother feel better about her only daughter having a baby "out of wedlock," as her mother put it. Donna went on to tell me that her father had threatened never to see her or her baby if she didn't marry the bum. But the moment Donna phoned from the hospital to say that the baby was born, they were both down there weeping through the nursery window, arguing over which grandparent was responsible for the baby's good looks.

I told Donna that I was really happy that everything had turned out well for her, but that, unfortunately, things hadn't gone so well for me. This was the first chance I had had to tell her that I had been through two miscarriages. I told her I was seriously considering giving up the idea of ever having a baby. I went on to say that John had really come around in the last few months. He had even pretended to look forward to "circle days." In fact he had been doing everything he knew how to make me feel better.

Donna listened patiently as I rambled on about how I could be happy in my thirties and forties without a baby if I had been happy in my twenties. I was sure of that, I said. Joyce Carol Oates had no children and she wrote a couple of books a year. If she had kids, she might be spending her days shopping and running car pools. Then I tried to think of another successful person who didn't have kids, but Donna's baby started crying. She broke in to say that she had to get off the phone and feed her baby. When she said "feed her," all my false bravado went down the drain. I hung up and cried.

As the weeks progressed, Donna phoned several

times to give support. She kept reminding me that if she could have a baby, I could have one too. She added that it was just a matter of time, and that I shouldn't give up after everything I had been through.

I was grateful for Donna's encouragement, but I still wasn't so sure I could take her advice and try again. I was thirty-four. I had already wasted two years thinking of nothing but becoming pregnant. I could continue doing this for another half a dozen years. But there were no guarantees that I'd end up having a baby. I could be forty with nothing to show for it, except a medicine chest full of empty Clomid bottles and a dresser drawer jammed with circled temperature charts. I told Donna that if I were ten years younger and there were no biological time clock breathing down my neck, perhaps I could spare the time and energy. There were even fleeting moments when I actually considered having my tubes tied so that I wouldn't be tempted to torture myself with further efforts to have a baby.

I tried explaining to Donna how painful that first miscarriage had been. But when the second arrived, I felt as if my entire body had been anesthetized to the pain. For weeks afterward I had to keep reminding myself what I had been through. Still I could feel nothing—no pain would register. I almost began to believe that my favorite proverb had been answered: do not pray for what you desire—pray to lose the desire.

Donna listened patiently as I went on to describe the feeling of numbness and how it lasted for several weeks before dissolving into a kind of hurt I didn't even know I was capable of feeling. It was silent and insidious and hung over me like a cloud for weeks.

As I continued describing the impact of the miscarriages, occasionally I stopped to make sure I wasn't getting too maudlin. Donna claimed that I wasn't, and that it was good I was getting it all out. Although Patsy had been my closer friend, she had never understood the way Donna did.

Patsy's genuine concern and willingness to listen had been a comfort. It was just that she found it difficult to grasp the psychological impact of my miscarriages. I tried explaining that, once I learned I was pregnant, it didn't matter if I were only five minutes pregnant or five months. The fact was that I was pregnant. And that was that.

Patsy attempted to console me by relating horror stories about how she had almost died when her first child was born. When I didn't react, she went on to say that it was touch-and-go with the second and third too. Her catastrophic childbirth stories only made me want to have a baby more.

When the birth stories didn't work, she tried a different tack. She told me how she had gone into a depression after auditioning for a major musical production—a production that could have turned her career around—and failing. Because I knew that Patsy was just trying to make me feel better about the miscarriages, I never mentioned that an intense desire to dance couldn't match an intense desire to have a baby. When a choreographer doesn't give you the part, it's one person's taste. But when you can't have a baby, it's nature who is not giving you the part. And when nature turns on you—*that* is the ultimate rejection slip.

During one of Donna's last calls, she told me that she had just read an interesting article in the local paper about an infertility support group: several couples who meet once a week to discuss their problems. My initial reaction was that it was probably like one of those California "rap-and-touch" sessions that had been popular in the sixties. I made it a point never to get involved in groups of that sort. The last group I had been affiliated with was the Blue Birds, a right-wing organization, in the second grade.

But the more I thought about that infertility support group, the more curious I became. Maybe they could offer some insight into my particular dilemma. I thought that since John had been coming around more and more, perhaps he might just be willing to give it a try.

But before I could even explain the idea behind the group, he simply said no.

"You're not listening," I said. "They might just help us cope better."

"We are not going to sit around with fifty strangers and discuss our sex life," he said.

"There aren't fifty."

"Whatever. A hundred voyeurs glaring at *me* while you rattle off our most private life as if you're reading off minutes of a meeting."

I tried telling him that they didn't discuss anything to do with circles. They discuss the psychological aspects of infertility. At least that's what I gathered from the article Donna read to me.

Then I began telling him what a few of the couples said in the interview.

"They sound perverted," John said. This was predictable.

I didn't press the issue. I had subjected him to enough mental and physical pressure in the past year. If he felt that adamant, I would back off. Besides, I wasn't so sure that even I wanted to go.

Six weeks later there was someplace that we both wanted to go. John was researching a story that would necessitate going to the remote jungles of New Guinea where a Stone Age tribe of headhunters live virtually untouched by the Western world. When John came to me with this news, he also gave me an option: I could either stay home and memorize my books on miscarriage, or I could accompany him on his assignment and research material for my own article.

I phoned Patsy to tell her about the trip and how ironic it was that their culture and art emphasized fertility. But Patsy seemed more interested in telling me how ironic it was that I wasn't pregnant. She reminded me that, if I had been, I certainly wouldn't be going off to any malaria-infested jungle to see the headhunters. I'd be home with my swollen feet jammed into a bucket of ice water watching "Bowling for Dollars."

Patsy had a point. I wondered how I would have felt if I had been pregnant and John had to go without me. At first I thought that even if I had been pregnant I could still make the trip. But then I discovered that it was necessary to take Cloroquine, malaria tablets, which have been linked to birth defects. For a split second I was actually relieved not to be pregnant. Then I felt guilty. Just days earlier I had been terribly despondent. I wondered if this erratic behavior was typical of the obsessed.

The day after we arrived home from our adventure, I could hardly wait to tell Patsy that the trip turned out to be as terrifying as I had hoped. I told her that when I spotted those Stone Age people with their plumes of feathers stuck in their hair, bones in their noses, and bodies covered in war paint, I didn't care if I *ever* got pregnant. All I wanted to do was to get the hell out of there with all my working parts, and with John's parts too.

After I was sure Patsy got the full impact of what I had been through, I invited her over to inspect the Asmat carving we brought back with us. She claimed not to be superstitious, but she still didn't want to get anywhere near a fertility statue. She said that with her luck she would end up pregnant with ten little headhunters.

But as it turned out, I was the one who ended up pregnant. For the third time in less than a year, I had a positive blood test. The third pregnancy came only four months after my last miscarriage. And it was a Clomid pregnancy, just as the other two had been. This convinced me more than ever that nature really did need that extra nudge. But even though it appeared that it was the Clomid that helped me to conceive, I was concerned that it might have also been the Clomid that had caused the miscarriages. I didn't want to be pessimistic, but nevertheless the thought haunted me to the point where the excitement of my pregnancy was dulled to a cautious optimism. I didn't tell the whole world this time: just a handful of friends, a few casual acquaintances, and whoever was listening when I accidentally mentioned it during a local TV interview about our trip.

During the first two months of my pregnancy, I had weekly Beta Sub Unit blood tests. The purpose of this test was to monitor the progesterone level, to make sure that there was an adequate amount to maintain the pregnancy. There was. When my pregnancy reached eleven weeks, one week longer than ever before, I began to relax to the point where I would carry my own groceries out to the car, though not before I made certain that the checker packed each bag as lightly as possible. Although my doctor had made a specific point of telling me to continue to do everything I did before I was pregnant, I still insisted on pampering myself. John more than willingly went along with this.

On my third prenatal visit came the big event: my doctor was to listen for the baby's heartbeat for the first time. As the nurse took my blood pressure, I bombarded her with questions: Is it normal to have no morning sickness? Why have I gained only five pounds? My stomach doesn't seem to be sticking out yet—is that normal? Why don't I crave weird food? I'm always tired; are you sure that's okay? Are you positive that the pregnancy test was accurate?

Before my questions got more paranoid, the nurse cut in. She politely but firmly told me that if I was to maintain any semblance of mental health, I would have to direct my energies toward more positive thoughts. Then she smiled softly and told me that she heard the doctor coming, and that I would soon hear my baby's heartbeat. When she said "your baby's heartbeat" it was the first time I believed that I was really pregnant.

Finally the doctor came in carrying what looked like a car battery with a long cord and microphone attached. He said it was called a Doppler Ultra-sound, and that I would be able to hear the baby's heartbeat over the amplification unit. As soon as he detected it, he would send the nurse out to get John so he could hear it too. I was suddenly glad that John was in the waiting room. At first I hadn't wanted him to drive me to the office. But he insisted, saying that he wanted to pick up a special book at the library. I knew that wasn't the truth. He wanted to be with me just in case there was no heartbeat.

Within moments the doctor placed the microphone on my abdomen. Out of nervousness I began talking, but he asked that I remain as quiet as possible so that he could locate the heartbeat. Almost as soon as he placed the microphone on my stomach, I heard a thump-thump-thump. Before I had a chance to get excited, he informed me that that was my heartbeat, not the baby's. I asked him what my heartbeat was doing down by my navel. He said that the Ultra-sound picks up the sound of moving fluid. And because he was directing the microphone down toward the large blood vessels in the uterus, it was picking up the sound of the blood being pumped by the heart through these vessels. The result was that I was actually hearing my own heartbeat.

Then he slid the microphone several inches lower and moved it in a circular motion. It seemed as if it was taking him an awfully long time. I began to get worried. All the while I had been checking his eyes for signs of bad news.

I was just getting ready to ask if everything was okay when I heard a quick thump-thump-thump. It was about twice as fast as my heartbeat. Then there was a fraction of total silence before my doctor shouted, "We did it! We have a baby!"

With that the nurse shouted exactly the same thing and went to get John.

I could not react. I lay there feeling somehow strangely detached from the situation, afraid to comment for fear I was dreaming or that the heartbeat might somehow be a mistake. When I saw John come into the examining room, I tried to tell him the news, but all that came out were tears.

For some reason my mind flashed back to the time when I was six years old. My parents had surprised me with a two-wheeler bicycle for Christmas. When I saw the bike with a big red ribbon around the handlebars, I didn't dare go over to it. I was afraid that it wasn't really for me, that it was too good to be true. So I stood there motionless before I ran up to my bedroom and cried.

Now, nearly thirty years later, I felt exactly the same way. But this time I wasn't alone. John was at my side. His eyes were a little watery. He held my hand and whispered, "We have our baby, Liz."

Suddenly I looked toward the door to see what all the commotion was about. My doctor was waving half the office staff in to listen to the heartbeat. They were all saying the same thing: "We have a baby." Even the new receptionist joined in.

That evening John phoned his youngest son, Judd, who was beginning his junior year at college. When Judd heard the news, all he requested was that it be a boy. Judd wanted a brother who could follow in his footsteps. I was glad that he was so enthusiastic. I was more than aware that older children often resent their father getting remarried and having younger children. If this had been the case, John would have had additional stress to cope with.

After we said goodbye to Judd, I phoned my parents to give them the news. As usual, the connection was bad. That was because they had half a dozen extensions. Everyone who lived there, plus those who were just visiting, would pick up the phone and listen. I didn't mind them listening if they would at least acknowledge their presence. But usually all I would hear was heavy breathing.

This time all the listeners acknowledged their presence. They all began talking at once. My mother was telling me that she would be coming up to help when the baby was born. My younger sister was saying that she'd be up too. My younger brother was arguing with my sister, reminding her that she would be in the middle of finals and that, anyway, she was afraid to fly. My sister's friend was on the phone telling me that her horse just had a baby colt. My father wasn't saying anything. I think he still had a nagging fear that I was going to dump the kid off when John and I went on one of our trips.

When my mother mentioned that she would buy the baby's layette, I told her to hold off on everything. I wasn't going to make any preparations for the baby until I had my amniocentesis test. That was scheduled to be during my eighteenth week of pregnancy, just six weeks away. Then before we hung up my mother added that the whole family would be coming up for the baby's christening, of course. The word *christening* conjured up memories of what Father O'Brien had told our second-grade class about baptism: "If a baby is not baptized it will never get to heaven. It won't go to hell. It will go to limbo." I took it that limbo was sort of like living in Akron the rest of your life.

CHAPTER
8

Amniocentesis

One month before my amniocentesis test, a brown manila envelope arrived from the Yale University School of Medicine, where I would be having my test. It contained information about the amniocentesis procedure.

Basically the letter said that, although amniocentesis is a proven technique for detecting chromosomal abnormalities, there is still no guarantee that the procedure will avoid damage to the mother or fetus. There is also a possibility that the test will result in a premature rupture of the membranes, causing a miscarriage. Studies in the United States and Canada show that the risk

101

of amniocentesis-related miscarriage is about a 1 in 200 chance. But at Yale the risk is considerably less—1 in 400.

The letter also stated that the attempt to get the amniotic fluid could be unsuccessful. This happens usually because it is too early in the pregnancy and there isn't enough amniotic fluid. If that is the case, another tap would be made a week or two later. There is also a small chance that, once they get the amniotic fluid, the cells will not grow, and a second test would be recommended to obtain more fluid with cells. The letter went on to say that there could be birth defects and mental retardation that remained undetected by the test. For this, there is a 1 in 30 chance. But what bothered me more than anything was the part about the amniocentesis causing a possible miscarriage.

After I read that letter over twice, I phoned the genetics department at Yale. Before I made any decision, I wanted to know what the chances of carrying a Down's Syndrome baby were for other age groups. I learned that a thirty-year-old has a 1 in 880 chance, whereas I at thirty-five years old, had a 1 in 370 chance. The risk goes up with age. At thirty-seven it is 1 in 220, at forty 1 in 110, and at forty-nine 1 in 12. Obviously, the higher the age, the more important amniocentesis is.

I thought back to when I was in my twenties. If I had read that same letter then, would I still have postponed having a baby? After considerable thought I came to the conclusion—yes. There might have been fewer physical risks then, but I would have had more mental stress. I used to have nightmares that I was pregnant and that my life was doomed. Now that I think about it, I wouldn't even have read anything about the medical risks of waiting to have children, because I simply was not interested in having any.

The fact was that I *had* waited until my mid-thirties. Apparently the risks were greater, but my mental state was better (before my fertility problems, that is). Since all life is a gamble, I was willing to take my chances, and the amniocentesis at least would reduce the risk to a minimum. John and I signed the "informed consent statement" that came with the letter and sent it back to Yale.

Our appointment was set for three days before Christmas. But when John looked out the window that day and saw that our car was buried in snow, he wanted to postpone the test. I insisted that we keep the appointment, because I was already seventeen and one-half weeks pregnant. The cut-off date for amniocentesis is twenty weeks, and with the holidays coming up I was afraid that I wouldn't get another appointment. Amniocentesis is only performed between the fourteenth and twentieth weeks of pregnancy. It is not done before fourteen weeks because there isn't enough amniotic fluid to spare the twelve to twenty milliliters needed for the fetal study. And it isn't done after twenty weeks because it takes a full month to culture the results. This would bring the woman up to twenty-four weeks of pregnancy, by which time the fetus is termed "viable." Abortions are only permitted after this time if there is a threat to the mother's life.

Our first stop was at the admissions office, where a woman took routine registration information and punched it into a computer. Then she handed me what looked like a plastic credit card along with a medical chart. She instructed us to proceed fifty yards up the glass corridor to the blood laboratory.

Once there, I had a blood test for alpha-fetaprotein. This was to screen for a condition known as spina bifida, an opening in the baby's brain, spinal column, and abdomen. Spina bifida affects one out of every one thousand births in the United States. It is a congenital abnormality of the child's nervous system that involves a failure of the brain and spine to fully develop, leaving the baby severely paralyzed and/or mentally retarded.

After we left the lab, we took an underground tunnel that led to the section of the hospital where the amniocentesis would be performed. As we walked through the tunnel, I wondered how women ever got through their pregnancies before these tests were available. In the last few weeks I had asked my mother that more than once. And more than once she had told me that when she was pregnant she wouldn't allow herself to think or read anything negative. That was the big difference between us. I read *everything* on pregnancy—the more negative it was the more I dwelled on it. In fact the last time I had spoken to my mother, I had read her a few of the dismal statistics, but before I even got into percentages, she hung up on me, only to call back several minutes later and insist on talking to John. She told him to throw away all of my "crazy" books.

But of course John didn't do anything of the sort. It's not that he thought it was a bad idea; rather, I had warned him that if he tossed the books in the trash, his Marlboros and my books would be fellow passengers on the way to the dump. In the last few months, I had cut out a half dozen or so articles on the harmful effects of secondhand cigarette smoke. But John counteracted my articles with specious advertising put out by the Tobacco Growers Association.

Worse than secondhand cigarette smoke is actually smoking. Studies have shown that smoking can result in prematurity, smaller babies, and even miscarriage. If a woman is a heavy smoker she has a two and one-half times greater chance of delivering a premature baby than a woman who does not smoke. In addition, smokers have a tendency to have babies of low birth weight, which may be a serious threat to the baby's life. There is also a link between heavy smoking and birth defects.

We emerged from the tunnel and made our way to Yale's perinatal unit, where we sat in a cramped hallway waiting for the genetic counselor. Across from us was a woman wearing a pair of jeans with the zipper about to pop. I felt a little envious of her very obvious bulge. I thought I could have really used something like that to go with the brand new maternity outfit I was wearing. Next to her was a guy who looked as if his name should have been Bruiser. Bruiser kept making a fist with one hand and punching it into the open palm of his other.

I couldn't be sure if he was nervous or just mad that his wife had made him miss a day's work. John had his own way of dealing with anxiety. He sat stone upright as if rigor mortis had set in.

Thirty minutes after Bruiser and his wife were led down the corridor to the amniocentesis room it was our turn to see the counselor. She was direct and efficient. She carefully reviewed everything that had been spelled out in the letter, stopping every so often to ask if we had any questions. Basically she wanted to make sure that we understood that there was a small chance that the amniocentesis would cause a miscarriage. She also stressed that the amniocentesis does not screen for all types of birth defects. In fact all pregnancies carried a 3 percent chance (1 in 30) of the occurrence of some type of serious birth defect that would not be detected by their testing. Once she was certain that we were well aware of those facts, she began to describe what I would be experiencing just minutes later.

At that point John started to excuse himself, saying that he had a weak stomach and that he would just wait in the hallway. I began explaining to the counselor that I realized the letter suggested husbands join their wives for the test, but that John could never do that. John was just sitting there nodding in agreement, encouraging me to elaborate on how he couldn't handle it the way he was sure other husbands could.

Evidently the counselor had heard all of this before. She was sympathetic, but not condescending. She merely told us that if John was that adamant he should by all means not stay for the test. But she did strongly suggest that he be with me for the Ultra-sound scan. The scan is done prior to the amniocentesis.

The Ultra-sound is a safe and painless technique for obtaining pictures of the fetus inside the uterus. This is done by sliding a stethescopelike instrument across the abdomen to pick up sound waves. The sound waves are then projected onto a televisionlike screen, producing an image that resembles a crude black and white TV picture. There are several reasons for using the Ultra-sound in conjunction with amniocentesis: to locate the best pocket of amniotic fluid; to avoid any possible injury to the fetus; to determine the exact age of the fetus; to see if it is growing normally; and to see if there is more than one fetus (although sometimes, if one fetus is directly behind another, it may appear that there is only one fetus).

Finally John halfheartedly agreed to stay for the Ultra-sound picture. But he made it clear that he would *not* be around for the needle work. On the way out of the counselor's office, she turned to John and said that it was just as well he wasn't staying for the entire procedure because even men who *were* enthusiastic often passed out. Bruiser had been one of those. As we walked down the corridor, there he was, lying on a stretcher semiconscious. His wife was pressing cold compresses to his forehead, trying to bring him around. John winced as we passed him.

After I put on a white smock and lay down on the steel table, a nurse rubbed gel on my abdomen. Then she turned off the lights and began sliding the scanner across my middle, pressing down firmly as she did so. That was the worst part of the test since, in order to obtain a clear picture, it was necessary to have a very full bladder.

I kept my eyes fixed on the small screen off to my left, waiting for my 4½-month-old baby's image to appear, hoping that there would be only *one*. All the while John was still acting jumpy. He kept reminding the nurses to be sure to let him know when it was time for him to leave. They kept reassuring him that the amniocentesis would not be performed until the doctor showed up. The doctor was the only one who could do the test, and he wasn't coming in until they located the exact position of the fetus.

After a few minutes of sliding the scanner from one end of my abdomen to the other, the nurse finally came to a gradual stop. Then the other nurse walked over to the screen, and they began consulting each other as to what they were seeing. I couldn't see anything that even remotely resembled a baby. It looked like just a bunch of wavy lines. Only seconds later she slid the scanner very slowly a quarter of an inch lower and held it firmly in place while the other nurse adjusted a knob below the screen.

At that very moment my baby came into focus. But it didn't look like what I had imagined. Even though we had been told exactly what to expect, I had not expected to see such a perfectly formed human being. I had thought that hearing the heartbeat at twelve weeks had been a thrill. But seeing my baby vigorously kicking its little arms and legs was as spectacular and unreal as the first moon landing.

By the time the image on the screen registered I had transported myself back to Cleveland in the fifties. My backyard to be exact. I was five years old playing with Cherry Preuss. We were pushing our doll carriages. I was telling Cherry that the moment I got married I was going to go to the hospital and get a baby who looked just like Tiny Tears. But Cherry said that I might not get a baby at all. Her aunt had never had a baby and that was why she was all shriveled and had a bird. I might just have to get a bird. I told her to mind her own fat business. I was getting a baby. She could get a bird. Now, as I watched my baby kick, stretch, and move its fingers in some sort of sign language, I wondered if I should send Cherry a birth announcement.

In addition to Cherry I would have to send Nima, our Sherpa friend from the Himalayas, a birth announcement too. Several times Nima had asked why I never had children. He said that it would be very good luck to have a baby in the house. Sherpas love children. In fact one of the worst sins a Sherpa can commit is to make a child cry. Nima once said that my age should not stop me from having a baby. His mother was also very, very old when she had his youngest brother. I asked how old "very, very old" was. He said she was twenty-eight, maybe twenty-nine.

When Nima referred to me as very old he was actually complimenting me. Sherpas don't have the age hang-ups Americans have. Sherpas believe that the older person is wiser and better than the younger person. This is because the older person has had more time on earth to do good deeds. And the more good deeds, the higher you go after you die.

"Look," the nurse said as she pointed toward the screen. "He's waving hello."

I was so excited that I forgot to look over toward John for his reaction. In fact, the only reason I took my eyes off the screen was to prevent John from squeezing my fingers off.

"It's a miracle. It is just a miracle. Nothing but a miracle," John was mumbling.

Although the nurses must have seen thousands of fetuses, they appeared as excited as we were. They took turns pointing out each time the baby moved to a different position, commenting on how active the fetus was.

John and I watched as one nurse measured the diameter of the baby's head. A metric scale was superimposed on the screen to reveal the diameter and to determine the exact age. According to the size of the head, my baby was eighteen and a half not seventeen and a half weeks old. But I told the nurse that the machine was wrong. I explained that I was positive about exactly when I had conceived, because I kept temperature charts and copious notes that month. When I said that, John squeezed the tips of my fingers. It was his way of letting me know that it wasn't the time or place to get into the fertility thing.

The nurse made a few minor adjustments on the

screen before taking a series of photos using some sort of polaroid camera that was part of the Ultra-sound machine. All but two of the black and white prints went to the doctor for his inspection. The remaining two were handed over to John. Later he would drag the photos out of his wallet to show our friends pictures of his "youngest."

A millisecond after the doctor entered, John was out of the testing room. And for a fleeting moment I actually considered doing the same. Until I came face to face with the doctor, I had no question that I would have the amniocentesis. It was an important test not only because of my maternal age, but also because of the correlation between John's paternal age and fetal abnormalities.

Now, as I lay watching my very own baby moving its fingers and toes, I thought about telling the doctor to forget it. I'd take my chances. I would be taking a 1 in 400 chance that this amniocentesis would result in a miscarriage. And a 1 in 30 chance that, even with the amniocentesis, I would still give birth to an abnormal baby. I thought, what if this test showed that I was one of the unfortunate women to be carrying a Down's Syndrome baby? Could I terminate this pregnancy at twenty-two and one-half weeks, knowing that in only a week and a half it would have a chance of surviving? I suddenly wished I hadn't even seen the baby on the screen.

My apprehension began to build even further when the doctor ran the scanner across my abdomen, trying to determine where the best pocket of amniotic fluid was. Once he located the spot, he somehow marked it in a way I couldn't quite see. Then the gel was wiped off, and an iodine solution was painted on. After that a green sterile drape was placed over the area.

Seconds later, he injected a local anesthetic in the vicinity of the marked spot. It felt as if I had been stung by a bee. But after ten seconds there was no pain. Before the doctor did the actual amniotic tap, he comforted me by saying that the needle would be no bigger than the kind used to withdraw blood from an arm. But when he added that it had to be long enough, of course, to penetrate the abdomen and uterus, I shut my eyes tightly and nodded. Then he asked that I remain perfectly still. When he said that, I became alarmed. I told him that I would try, but what would happen if the sensation of the needle made me flinch involuntarily? He said that there would be no painful sensation. Most patients feel only slight pressure as the needle is inserted into the uterus.

At that I turned my head away from him, closed my eyes, and waited for the needle to enter. But I never felt the needle. In fact if the nurse hadn't said halfway through the three-minute procedure that good, clean amniotic fluid was filling the syringe, I would never have known that the test had begun. As soon as the doctor had extracted twenty cubic centimeters, the needle was withdrawn. The syringe was immediately closed, labeled, and sent to the laboratory. I would find out the results in four weeks.

By the time we had left Yale, it was nearly noon. The snow had stopped. John drove well under the speed limit, avoiding all the potholes. The last thing the nurses said was that I should be sure to take it easy the rest of the day. I took their advice, staying in bed the rest of the day and half of the next. By the following afternoon I felt certain that I was on safe ground. If anything was going to happen, it would have already. Besides, I had things to do. We were having friends in for Christmas brunch. They were strays as we were, with families all somewhere else.

John had surprised me and put up our tree. He didn't want me straining myself by reaching, even though the tree was less than three feet tall and artificial. At first glance, the tree looked wonderful, but on closer inspection all the bulbs were lumped together. There weren't any on the back of the tree. I immediately rearranged them. Pleased with my design, I backed up to admire the finished tree, failed to notice that our large standard poodle was sleeping at my heels, and landed flat on my back.

John, in his office, heard only the dog's screech and my scream. He ran down the stairs and practically carried me to the sofa. Then he started toward the phone to call the doctor. I told him not to. I was okay; it was just the suddenness that had frightened me. Pregnant women fall off horses and down flights of stairs all the time, and nothing ever happens. But what kept flashing through my mind was what had happened to John's sister. In her third month of pregnancy, she had fallen on ice and miscarried the next day. I lay on the sofa scared to death.

I must have stayed there for at least two hours—waiting for the worst to happen. But it never did. When I finally got up, I was fine. I didn't have an ache or pain anywhere. But around three in the morning I woke up with an excruciating pain on my right side near my ovary. Every five minutes or so it would come and go. This pattern continued about four hours and I was sure this was it. At seven o'clock I phoned the doctor. He said I should come right down to his office.

The minute we stepped into the waiting room, the nurse took me in to be examined. Moments later, my doctor came in carrying the Ultra-sound machine to listen for the baby's heartbeat. It was there—loud and clear. It was quite extraordinary how just hearing my baby's heartbeat diminished the pain.

The doctor said that apparently I had pulled a muscle during the backflip, but it should go away in a few days. He reassured me that everything was normal. On my way out, he suggested that for the next five months I avoid walking backward.

Waiting for the Test Results

Christmas had come and gone. It was now early January. John was preparing to leave on a TV and radio tour for his latest book. I was in the middle of writing about Nima and the cultural shock of his leaving the Himalayas to come to Connecticut. And we were both more than a little anxious waiting for the pending amniocentesis results. John was only anxious because I made him that way. But I couldn't help myself. In the previous week, I had just begun to feel the baby move, which was more exciting than hearing the heartbeat or even seeing the baby in action on the Ultra-sound screen.

The reason the amniocentesis results took four weeks was because the cells had to grow and reproduce. Once the vial of amniotic fluid arrives at the laboratory it is spun in a centrifuge to separate the cells from the fluid. These cells are placed in an incubator and cultured for about a month. If the lab technician notices that the cells are not growing, another amniotic tap must be performed. As soon as there is adequate cell growth, the cells are washed in a solution that enlarges the chromosomes, making them easy to view under a microscope. Finally, the chromosomes are photographed. The photos are then blown up, cut out and arranged into a karyotype, which shows the actual imprint of the image of the chromosomes. The karyotype is analyzed by the doctor, who then interprets the results. Included in the results is the baby's sex. Some couples choose not to be told what their baby's sex will be. We were one of those couples. John and I figured that since everything leading up to and including the amniocentesis had been reduced to a science, we would have an old-fashioned birth and end up surprised.

There was no way I could wait for the four weeks required to learn the results of the culture. After only two, I phoned just in case there was any news. And I was glad that I did. Although they had no information on the chromosomes, they did say that the alpha-fetaprotein blood test for spina bifida was normal.

Once I learned that, I was told to call back in two weeks for the chromosome results. But I was so edgy, probably because of the two miscarriages still fresh in my mind, that I called back after only one week. I rationalized this behavior by telling myself that I had been through more than my share, and I had every right to make a nuisance of myself.

I dialed the genetics department hoping that the same woman would not answer. The woman had been so accommodating the first time, and I didn't want to wear out my welcome. Whoever it was who answered seemed very understanding when I explained about the two miscarriages and how totally paranoid I was that there would be something wrong. But she still had no further information. I was told to wait *at least* another week.

When I hung up I had every intention of waiting an extra week, but only four days later I had an uncontrollable urge to phone back.

This time I recognized the woman's voice. When I reluctantly gave her my name there was a lull before she said that if I would hang on a moment she would phone the lab on the other line. Several minutes later, she came back on the line to report that everything appeared to be growing just fine. It's just a matter of time before getting some more cells to examine. Then she told me to call back in a week.

But I cut the week three days short and gave them another ring. Still no results. Two days later I called again. No luck. I waited twenty-four hours and called back. By this time they must have thought I was dead from the neck up. But at least there was some news. I was told that they had cultured seven out of twenty cells.

They all looked good, and they should have all the cells cultured by the end of the following week.

When she said "the end of the following week," I got miffed. I told the woman that that would make it five weeks to find out the results, not four as the letter stated. She explained that they had a backlog of patients and the ones who were farther along in their pregnancies took priority. I didn't tell the woman that I really couldn't sympathize with their backlog problem. However, I did make it clear that another week's wait would psychologically finish me off. In seven days I would be nearly twenty-three weeks pregnant—only one week away from the time the fetus would be termed viable and abortion illegal. As it was, I was carrying an almost completely formed human being. If I had to wait seven more days and the worst were confirmed, I might not be able to go ahead with an abortion. All she said in reply was that she understood how I felt, but I would still have to wait my turn.

I hung up, phoned my own doctor, and explained the situation. When he heard my voice change to a high-pitched whine, he promised to call the laboratory and see what additional information was available. Later that afternoon he phoned back and told me exactly what they had already said. No final results could be given out until a few more cells had been cultured. He reassured me that there was no problem, there were no secrets being kept from me, and that it was just a matter of policy. I should stop worrying. But I would continue to worry until I got the final word.

Six days later, I received a phone call from the genetics department.

"Mrs. Fuller," the voice on the other end of the line said.

"Yes."

"Yale calling with your amniocentesis results."

I knew that everything had to be okay. The letter had specifically stated that if anything were wrong my own doctor would call.

"You have forty-six chromosomes. There is no breakage. Everything appears to be normal. And you have XY chromosomes, which indicate a baby bo—"

I let out a yelp. "No. No. Don't tell me." But it was too late. I had already heard the "bo," and it was obvious that I was having a boy.

While I was recovering from the sudden shock, the woman was apologizing profusely for her accidental slip. This was the first time anything like this had ever happened to her and she was extremely sorry.

It took some time to digest this news before I found the words to say that it really didn't matter anyway. As long as the baby was okay, that's all that counted. I was certain my husband would feel the same.

The moment John had heard the animal sound coming from my office, he lunged up the stairs, naturally assuming that it was Yale with bad news. John was so relieved to learn that the amniocentesis was normal, he barely realized that we were having a boy. It wasn't until after I hung up that John commented. And then it was just to say that he had known from the Ultra-sound picture that it was a boy. He claimed that the shoulders were too square for a girl. John immediately grabbed the phone to call Judd at college, and I knew that he was thrilled. I had no preference, but once I found out, I told John that I had always wanted a boy for our *first* child. John did not even dignify that with a comment.

I had promised Patsy that I would call her the moment I heard from Yale. I made that same promise to Donna and my mother. But since I had upset Patsy the most, I called her first. In the previous few days I had done nothing but phone her to share my paranoid fears.

Patsy no sooner learned that everything was okay than she started on those horrible childbirth stories again. She added firm warnings that I *must* be prepared for all types of labor complications. She claimed that she wasn't trying to frighten me, but if I was not informed I could very well end up the way she had.

Patsy was referring to her twenty years of finely tuned abdominal muscles that had been sliced up in a five-minute emergency cesarean section. Patsy said that the doctor hadn't even taken into consideration that she was a professional dancer. He butchered her up so badly that she never danced again.

I felt Patsy had a legitimate reason for her birth hangup, but I told her that she didn't have to be concerned about me. I intended to take a prepared childbirth course.

Just then Donal picked up the extension and overpowered both of us with a bit of George Bernard Shaw.

Donal was still in his Shavian phase, which meant that he was never at a loss for an apropos Shaw anecdote. He recalled that Shaw had been at a dinner party seated next to a young society woman who began telling Shaw and half the dinner table that she couldn't decide whether she wanted to be burdened with children or not. Donal said that when Shaw had had his fill of the prattle, he turned to the woman and said: "Madame, nature does not care what you feel or want. Nature wants the child."

Whenever Donal related an anecdote he went on to analyze it to death, always ending up with his own interpretation. Donal figured that what Shaw meant by "Nature wants the child" was that the life force—for both female and male—was so powerful that it made personal preferences in decisions of whether or not to have children totally irrelevant.

I told Donal that I doubted that the paternal urge was as strong as the maternal. I cited my own case as an example. I did have to admit that ever since John had seen the baby on the Ultra-sound screen he hadn't brought up the $90,000 it would take for college. But given a choice, he would have preferred no baby at all. John had repeatedly said that he could have lived quite contentedly without kids. Although he was always quick to add that, as long as he had three kids, he loved them.

Donal said that this supported Shaw's point exactly. If John or any man had been that adamant about not having them, there would not have been any children. Donal's voice was hitting about ten on the Richter scale as he went on to argue that there was no way a woman could coerce a man into having children. If a man were absolutely opposed to it, he would either leave the situation or become impotent. I broke in to remind Donal that with modern birth control methods a man could have a child without wanting one. How would he know if the woman had stopped taking the pill? I'm not sure Donal took that point in. He just continued to say that at the core of our being there is that irrefutable life force perpetuating the human race. Just because we have relatively sophisticated minds, nature lets neither man nor woman off the hook. Then I thought Donal was going to split his lungs and our ear drums when he bellowed out, "Nature wants the child."

Patsy piped in and told Donal to clamp it—he was becoming too loud and too repetitive. But Donal kept right on going. He continued to say how he personally had had the paternal urge even before he married Patsy. Finally Patsy made herself heard on the extension. "Donal, you've made your bloody point!" With that, Donal signed off. But he got back on several moments later with one final George Bernard Shaw quote: "There is one experience that no woman has ever regretted, and that experience is motherhood. Celibacy for a woman is *il gran rifuto*—the greatest refusal of her destiny, of the purpose in life which comes before all personal considerations: the replacing of the dead by the living."

That evening John and I had dinner out to celebrate. At least it started off as a celebration. I told John that for the first time since the workup I felt truly relaxed, and for the next four months I was going to luxuriate in my pregnancy, allowing no negative thoughts to enter my mind. From here on in, nothing could possibly go wrong—I was sure of that. John picked up his martini and clicked it against my glass of club soda. I would have preferred to be toasting with a bottle of dry white wine. But in recent weeks the newspapers and magazines had been filled with warnings about the hazards of alcohol, caffeine, cigarettes, aspirin and other drugs. The general consensus seemed to be that everything the mother eats or drinks can be expected to reach the fetus minutes later.

As we ate dinner I began telling John how well prepared *we* were going to be for labor and birth. When I said "we," John asked what I meant. It was at this point that the tone of the evening changed.

I explained to John that we would have to think about a prepared childbirth course to get us through the labor and birth of our son. Before I ever got to the importance of "parent bonding" in the first few minutes of the baby's life, he simply said, "No go." He couldn't even discuss the subject without getting light-headed.

Since I didn't want to ruin the evening, I said that we would talk about it later, and I changed the subject. I asked him what he thought about the name Christopher. Without answering, he said that I might just as well forget about dragging him to one of those ridiculous classes with pubescent couples learning how to "parent bond." When John said "pubescent" it became apparent that he was worried that he'd look out of place or, for that matter, that both of us would. I reassured him by telling him that Donna had taken the course and in her particular class half of the couples were in their late thirties or early forties. I told John that two of the husbands had been in their sixties—a small exaggeration.

John said that he had once seen a cow give birth and the memory had never left him. He claimed that even today, whenever he thinks of that heifer moaning, he becomes so nauseated he can't finish eating. I tried explaining to him that that was because he didn't love the cow. Besides, he had been unprepared for what happened. You're always frightened when you don't know what to expect. With the childbirth classes, the husband has an active part in the delivery. But the more I tried to convince him, the more stubborn he became. Finally I told him to forget it. I would go alone.

Before I decided on what prepared childbirth class I would go to, I checked with Donna. But when Donna heard that I would be going without John, she said that she didn't recommend her particular class. She had been the only one in the class without a husband, and since the whole idea is based on couples sharing the birth experience, Donna's instructor had been thrown off balance. Donna got up to introduce herself to the class without mentioning her special status of being a "single mother." The instructor jumped to the conclusion that her husband worked evenings, and announced it to the class. Donna, who enjoyed shock value, promptly set the record straight: she had no husband. From that moment on, Donna felt she was resented by the instructor. But I wondered how much of this was Donna's own paranoia.

Since Donna seemed certain that my being without a husband would throw the instructor off, I decided to look for a class that could handle the situation. As it turned out, my doctor had mentioned on my sixth prenatal visit that his former nurse was teaching prepared childbirth two nights a week at his office. I had known and liked her from my early workup days.

When I returned home I phoned her and explained about John's queasy stomach and said that I would have to take the course without him. She said that that was no problem. In the class that had just ended, two women had been without their husbands. One woman started off with her husband, but after the second class he dropped out because of Monday night football.

The moment John learned that he was no longer needed he compromised. He would come to the classes, and maybe into the labor room for a few minutes. But he would not even peek into the delivery room.

10

Prepared Childbirth

On the thirtieth week of my pregnancy, John drove as slowly as he could to the doctor's office for that first lesson. We had been in the car only minutes before John began acting the martyr, reminding me that he was giving up the Stanley Cup playoffs on TV, something he had waited for all year.

As we got out of the car, I mentioned to John that in just two and a half months we would be headed down the road to the hospital. Then he would be glad he had come with me to the classes. John said that he would be the judge of that. He helped me up the stairs leading to the office, warning me all the while to watch for icy spots.

There were a total of six couples arranged on love seats scattered throughout the waiting room. The instructor was sitting on a chair facing the very expectant parents. Half of them looked like they were in their twenties, half of them in their thirties, and one husband looked like he was in his early fifties. John sat next to him. I squeezed between John and a young woman wearing a sweatshirt that said "Baby Under Construction." She looked even more pregnant than I did.

By the time I reached my seventh month, I had gone from looking only passably pregnant to looking like Bozo the tipping clown. But the larger I became, the more I enjoyed it. I loved every moment, even the terrible indigestion that comes with pregnancy. I had to keep reminding myself that pregnancy is not a final condition—pregnancies end with babies.

I don't know why I wanted to continue in the limbo state. Perhaps it was because it took me so long to get pregnant that I just wanted, selfishly, to keep my baby tucked inside, feeling it kick and move forever. But of course that was impossible. Maybe I was just afraid of the responsibility. Or I feared being a rotten mother. Or losing my self-identity. Just days earlier my mother had phoned and asked how my book on our Himalayan trek was coming. I told her I was halfway through it, and that I would finish it after the baby came.

I started to tell her how I intended to sct up my

office like a nursery, but she didn't let me finish. She said that I may as well just forget doing anything else until the baby started school. I couldn't believe she had really said that. I told her that I had no intention of changing my life style and that having babies today was not like having them thirty-five years ago. It was no longer necessary to compromise your career for a baby. Babies can adapt quite well. All she said in response was, "You'll see."

That "you'll see" haunted me for days afterward. I also thought a lot about what Barbara had said so many months earlier: "What if in ten years you wake up and realize you hate kids?" What if both my mother and Barbara were right? Suppose I gave the baby the best years of my life and the kid grew up to hate me, or vice versa. I didn't share these black thoughts with anyone—except Patsy. And I only shared them with Patsy because she noticed that something had been bothering me.

I didn't exactly come out and tell Patsy I was afraid I might not love my baby. I merely asked her when maternal love was supposed to come—before or after the baby was born? Patsy asked what my books had to say on the subject. I told her that, in all the books I had read, there was not a single thing on maternal love—just on postpartum depression. She didn't even acknowledge my attempt at humor.

Instead she said that we Americans have some ridiculous conception that love is supposed to be the way it is shown in the Coca-Cola commercials: California blondes and bubbly smiles. Love is not teenage bliss—

love is a bag full of emotions. Patsy said that if I wanted to know what real love is I should just wait until my kid comes home from grade school with a note saying that he hasn't done his homework in a month and he gives you every reason from Istanbul crud to Dengue fever. First you'll want to kill him. Then you'll want to kill yourself for wanting to kill him. That, she said, was love. Patsy went on to say that the humorist Dorothy Parker summed up love better than Freud: "They came and told me all your faults—they told them by the score. But what they didn't know was your faults just made me love you more."

While all this was going on in my mind, I hardly realized that the instructor was passing out the childbirth preparation manuals. After each couple had a manual, the instructor asked that we take turns introducing ourselves to the group.

The introductions began with a tall man dressed in a dark, pin-striped suit. He seemed not to know why he was there. Finally he said that his wife had phoned him at the office several hours earlier and told him not to be late and not to drink in the train's bar car. Then he gave a nervous chuckle. His attractive blonde wife playfully argued that he had known about the class for weeks. Again he gave a nervous laugh and put his long arm around her, pulling her near.

The couple next to them were from Pakistan. The wife spoke little English, so her husband gave their names. But he must have misunderstood the question. He said that the reason they were at the class was that it was close to their home. The instructor smiled and nodded that it was my turn. I told the group that I wanted to see my baby being born and not be all drugged up and in pain when I did so. I didn't mention the other reason: that my friend Patsy had made me so paranoid about the birth process. Then the instructor looked toward John, indicating it was his turn.

John never said why he was there. Instead he told the instructor that the moment she got out the color slides showing the actual birth process, he would have to wait in the car. Everyone laughed except John. The man next to John, the one who looked around fifty, immediately added that he couldn't take the slides either. He elbowed John and said that they would both go out for a cigarette when the slides were shown. There seemed to be an instant camaraderie between them. His wife rolled her eyes in a mood of indifference. She went on to say that they had two teenage children who had been born without the benefit of prepared childbirth, and so they wanted to do it with their last. When she said "their last," the husband again elbowed John and mumbled that it had better be the last.

The last couple to introduce themselves were the youngest. They both said exactly the same thing at exactly the same time. They wanted to share the entire birth experience of their baby. I assumed they had been married two minutes.

During that first class we learned that the course was based on the Lamaze method, named after the French obstetrician Dr. Fernand Lamaze. Dr. Lamaze developed his method after studying the theories of I. P. Pavol, a Russian neurologist who had built on the conditioned-reflex theories of Ivan Pavlov.

Pavol did not believe drugs were necessary to alleviate labor pains. He felt that, through intense psychological and physical education, the myths of painful childbirth could be destroyed. Dr. Lamaze adapted Pavol's method and began a program in France called "Childbirth without Pain." By utilizing specific breathing and relaxing exercises, Lamaze believed that painless childbirth could be achieved. The program included the husband as an integral part of the entire process, beginning with the first stages of labor and ending with the birth of the baby.

Our instructor told us that this course was based on a modified Lamaze method. It had been carefully outlined in a manual put together by two specialists named Patricia Lawson and Fredda Simon. Before we even opened the booklet, she asked that we substitute the words *labor contraction* for *uterine pain*. Just as Pavlov conditioned his dogs to respond to the bell by salivating, we were going to be conditioned to respond to a contraction by relaxing our muscles through a series of breathing exercises. These breathing techniques were a tool to distract our minds from the discomfort of the contractions.

Over the next five lessons we would learn exactly what was happening during each step of labor, and how to participate most effectively throughout the various stages. In essence we would be controlling the discomfort by positively working with, instead of against, the labor. I suddenly wished Patsy was in the class. Maybe then she would believe that we could be in control of our own bodies during labor and delivery. Once I had asked her why she hadn't taken a similar type of course. She had said that when she went to the hospital for her three children, prepared childbirth meant you brought your own boiled water.

By the end of the two-hour session we had practiced slow chest breathing, shallow upper-chest breathing, accelerated-decelerated breathing, transition breathing (known as "pant-blow"), and choo-choo breathing. All of this was articulated in the manual by such terms as "hah-hah, hah-hee" or "hah-hah, hah-phff" or simply "hah-phff, hah-phff."

While the women simulated mock contractions in practicing these different breathing patterns, the husbands were busy too. They were acting as coaches, counting down on our breathing, and even doing rhythmic stroking of our backs and necks. During these exercises John was mildly annoying. He interrupted the class three times. Once he asked the couple who appeared to be from India if all this wasn't straight out of a Hindu handbook, with the self-hypnosis and the yogalike breathing. The man replied rather stiffly that they were Moslems from Pakistan and knew nothing about Indian lore. The two other times John stopped the class he did so to ask whether a local anesthetic would be available in case my pain got too severe. Both times the instructor asked John to *please* not refer to the word *pain*. Then she reminded all of us that prepared childbirth did *not* mean that we couldn't have drugs. If we felt we needed something to reduce the discomfort we should by all means have something. It would not mean that we had failed. The goal of Lamaze was to have a healthy, safe delivery.

Just before the two-hour session was dismissed we were reminded to bring a pillow the following week for the relaxation exercises. But we never made that second Lamaze class. John had to make a short trip to Mexico to gather last-minute research. Since it would be the last time John and I would be exclusively together, I decided to go along. At first John thought I should stay home. He said that he didn't know anything about the small town where he would be interviewing. There might not be a hospital or a doctor for miles. But in the end I went anyway.

Now that I look back, I think the reason I went was not so much that I wanted to drag around hot, muggy streets in my seventh month as that I wanted to make a statement: my life was not going to change. I could be pregnant, have a baby, and continue just as I always had.

Fortunately my statement did not backfire. We made it back safe and sound and in time for the third Lamaze class. During the next four sessions we learned everything about labor and then some. Labor is divided into three stages. The first stage begins when the uterus contracts, causing the cervix (the entryway to the uterus) to dilate. The cervix slowly widens from the width of a toothpick to the size of a baseball, ten centimeters.

In beginning labor, the uterine contractions are infrequent, short in duration, and mild; they feel more like menstrual cramps. At this stage they are five minutes or more apart and last for thirty to forty-five seconds. During this part of labor we were to use a slow chest breathing exercise at the start of each contraction. We would begin by focusing our eyes on an object in the room in order to enhance concentration. Once our eyes were fixed we were to take a "deep cleansing breath," which is simply Lamaze terminology for a deep breath through the nose and out the mouth. This is supposed to aid in relaxation and also provide an exchange of oxygen.

Then we would begin a slow, deliberate inhalation through the nose, concentrating on expanding the chest, followed by a controlled exhalation through slightly parted lips. This is done six to nine times per minute, ending with another "deep cleansing breath." While we would be doing the rhythmic breathing our husbands, who are called coaches, were to keep time, calling out every fifteen seconds how much time is left for the sixty-second contraction.

I wasn't so sure that I would like John being my coach during the real thing. As it was, all through the practice sessions he kept breaking my concentration to correct my pattern of breathing. The instructor even told

John that *she* thought I had it right. But John argued that I was still taking in air through my mouth instead of my nose. He insisted that the instructor hold her hand next to my mouth to check the intake of air.

Toward the end of that first stage of labor, the cervix dilates from around three centimeters (about the size of a Ping-Pong ball) to around seven to ten. The contractions increase in frequency, intensity, and duration. They may now occur every two minutes and continue for nearly a minute. This is called transition—the most difficult part of labor. Because the baby is pressing against a partially dilated cervix, there is a tremendous feeling of pressure accompanied by a strong urge to push. But pushing before full dilation is a waste of energy and could cause damage to the cervix. It is at this time that the breathing is so important. During transition we would be using a pant-blow technique, three shallow breaths through the mouth followed by a blow. To resist the urge to push we would use one shallow breath followed by a blow. Using this type of breathing would make it difficult to push, which must not be done before full dilation.

The second stage of labor begins after transition, when the cervix is fully dilated to the size of a baseball. The cervix can now be thought of as a door that the baby eventually will pass through. During this stage of labor, the contractions are usually not as intense because the baby is no longer forced against a partially opened cervix. This second stage of labor is actually easier because you can now follow your urge and begin pushing. The force of the push counteracts the strong contraction and brings a certain amount of relief.

The method we practiced in the class for pushing was first to lean back on our elbows in a semipropped position with knees bent. We then placed our hands under the knees, firmly grasping the thighs. As the simulated contraction began, we took two deep cleansing breaths. Then we inhaled for a third time and, while still holding the breath, placed our chins on our chests and began contracting our abdominal muscles and directing the pushing down and out. We were told to hold the breath and push as long as possible. The most effective pushes were the long steady ones. When we needed another breath, we moved our head back, exhaled, quickly inhaled, placed our chin back on our chest, and began pushing again. This stage of labor lasts from a half hour to two hours or more, ending only with the birth of the baby.

All through this pushing stage the husbands had specific tasks. The manual outlined everything, from directing the coaches to support our heads and shoulders to reminding them not to wander around the delivery room. But I didn't have to worry about John wandering around any delivery room. At the last Lamaze class, John's parting words to the instructor were that he would go no further than the labor room, and then he would only stay there for the slow chest breathing. The moment I moved into transition breathing, he said emphatically, he would move to the father's waiting room.

I think it was the childbirth slides that confirmed John's original fears. John sat through the normal delivery slide show, but went out to the parking lot for the cesarean delivery. I wished he had left for both. He complained all the way through the slides, saying that there was no reason to show extreme close-ups—we could have easily gotten the idea with camera long shots.

The final stage of labor comes after the baby is born when the placenta is delivered. This usually happens after a few postdelivery contractions. The placenta is what the baby has lived and fed off for the previous nine months.

On the last evening of class our instructor summed up the purpose of the course. She said it was to alert us to exactly what would happen during each phase of labor. We could then use the specific breathing exercises to work with the labor and not against it. By working positively with the contractions, we would be controlling the discomfort—keeping the use of drugs down to a minimum, or even discovering that we could do without medication.

However, our instructor pointed out that there could be situations where drugs are needed to ensure a safe, healthy delivery. Prepared childbirth did not mean having a baby totally without drugs. They could be used with discretion under the direction of the doctor. This would not mean that we had failed.

All of this sounded very exalted. But I was curious as to whether these breathing exercises, which sounded so great now, would really work when the time came.

Would I remember to do the slow chest breathing in the first part of labor? Or would I panic and do the pant-blow until I hyperventilated? Or would I forget all the breathing and scream for the strongest pain killer I could get?

But I wouldn't have to worry about that for the moment anyway. I had a full five weeks to rehearse everything from the hah-hah to the choo-choo breathing. By the time I went into labor, I would know the material cold. At least that is what I told Patsy the afternoon she dropped by with diet zucchini cake from the local health food store. I felt that the cake was simply another way of saying, "Lay off the sugar."

As the cake exchanged hands, she reminded me not to eat it all in one sitting. She warned that I had already gone from 105 to 141 pounds, and I still had five weeks left. I would never squeeze back into my suede jeans, and I may as well just pass them along to her now. And worse than that, my being overweight could lead to a complicated delivery. When she brought that up, I told her as diplomatically as I could to knock off the scare tactics. Just because she had had three dreadful delivery experiences, she really shouldn't dump her neurotic fears on me.

I told her that my doctor hadn't said a word about my weight gain, probably because I was too thin to begin with. In fact he had once said that he was no longer quick to put women on diets in order to keep them under a twenty-four-pound weight gain. In the past, a woman's weight was carefully controlled, and this often led to a lack of proper nutrition, resulting in low birth weight babies. And babies born under six pounds were usually not as healthy as the ones who weighed seven pounds and over. However, the doctor did add that if a woman was overweight at the start of her pregnancy and she went on to gain more than necessary her weight would be carefully monitored.

I asked why a twenty-four-pound weight gain was agreed on as the norm. He told me that the average baby weighs roughly seven to eight pounds; the placenta, one; the amniotic fluid, two; the increased weight of the uterus, two; the increased weight of the breast tissue, two; the increased blood volume, three; and excess water and fat, six. All this adds up to twenty-three pounds—the necessary weight gain needed to provide good nutrition to the mother and the developing fetus.

But Patsy didn't seem to be listening. She was too busy fumbling through a carton that my mother had just sent. It contained the baby's layette, complete with T-shirts, nightgowns, sweaters, terry cloth jumpsuits, towels, washcloths, receiving blankets, coming-home suit with matching shawl, bonnets, booties, burp rags, cloth diapers, rubber pants, crib sheets, mattress pads, a denim baby carrier that you wear like a pouch, a down blanket, a pillow, and a brush and comb set. All of this was topped off with two nightgowns, a bathrobe, and slippers for me. There was also a written sheet of instructions:

Things to pack for the hospital:
powder blue coming home suit with blue and white knit

shawl and two T-shirts. I got you cloth diapers, but you may want to use Pampers? Make sure you take shawl— even if it's a hot day. For yourself, I hope you like the nightgowns. I got the simplest I could find. Your sister picked out the pink and yellow. I know you hate pink, but dark colors are not right for when you have a baby. I got you slippers so you don't pack those crummy rubber shower shoes. Your father's worried about the pillow and blanket near the baby. Use the pillow just for decoration. Talk to you Sunday.

After Patsy read that note, she recalled what happened when she had her first baby. Her mother had come to the hospital with a pink nightgown and matching pink hair ribbon. Patsy had been doubled over in excruciating pain from the cesarean, and at the same time her mother had tried to tie a pink satin ribbon around her stringy hair. I quickly changed the subject before she began to elaborate.

I told Patsy that ever since the box of baby clothes had arrived, I no longer had a desire to remain pregnant forever. Just seeing that little coming-home suit with a duck on it made me wish I had the baby in my arms now. I thought that the ideal length of time to be pregnant would be eight months, not nine, and that these last five weeks would be the longest in my life. Patsy said they would be the longest in her life too. Before she left she said that I had better not have that baby before the showers.

There were two showers planned, although I had insisted on only one. My friends claimed that over the past three years too many of them had become personally involved in this pregnancy, and they all wanted to be included when it finally came to an end. Patsy said that the showers were more or less celebrations to mark the last time they would be forced to hear about my pregnancy.

One shower came and went. I now had only the month-plus to wait, with a nursery full of stuffed animals, mobiles, toys, and baby clothes to keep me company. John was more than solicitous in helping me maneuver around the house, even assisting with the meals.

Then on April 29 we phoned Judd at college to wish him a happy twenty-first birthday. In between telling us about the bash planned in his honor at the Chi Phi house, Judd said that he hoped the baby came a week late so that he would be finished with finals and home for summer break. I told Judd that I was *sure* the baby would be at least a week late. After we hung up, John went to the oven and took out the chicken he had prepared, and we sat down to watch the evening news.

Labor and Delivery

I had just taken my first bite of a slightly undercooked chicken breast when I became unmistakably aware that the amniotic sac had broken. When I told John about it, he immediately broke out in the panic I was trying to keep in. He took me by the arm and started to lead me over toward the bed, where I could lie down. I told him there wasn't time to lie down. I had to pack my suitcase for the hospital. Then I asked him to please lower his voice and get that weird look out of his eyes. For some reason, I was remarkably collected.

The instructor's words kept going through my mind:

"If the amniotic sac ruptures while you are at home, labor may start at any moment. Contact the doctor." I did. He said that I should come right down to the hospital where he would meet me in the labor room. When he said "labor room," I lost my initial calm. I told him that I couldn't be going into labor. I still had another four and a half weeks left. What would happen to my baby? He said that both the baby and I would be just fine and that he would talk to me further once we got there.

I hung up and began tossing nightgowns, bathrobes, slippers, a hair dryer, shampoo, the two infant T-shirts, and the blue coming-home suit in my red rucksack. Within minutes we were on the parkway headed toward the hospital. Nothing happened the way I had planned it. We hadn't even decided whether we would call the baby Christopher or Colin.

During the half-hour drive to the hospital we hardly spoke. When we did, it was only for John to check whether my labor pains had begun. I kept telling him that they hadn't, and reminded him that he was supposed to call them "contractions" instead of pains. But he continued to refer to them as pains all the way to the hospital and into the labor room.

It was a no-frill labor room. There was just a clock, a lamp, a chair, curtains, a bed, and a nurse with the firmness of a drill sergeant. Before I changed into my hospital gown, I realized that I hadn't called Patsy. I asked the nurse if I could first use the phone to call my friend. Without answering, she narrowed her eyes and told me to put the gown on and get into bed. Moments later the resident doctor appeared.

Meanwhile, John had gone out to finish parking the car. He had barreled into the emergency entrance as if I had been in the choo-choo breathing stage of labor. The security officer had reluctantly agreed to let him leave the car half up on the curb at an angle until he had deposited me in the labor room.

The resident doctor said that I was only a fingertip dilated (full dilation is five finger widths), and that he was going to have the nurse hook me up to a machine that would monitor the baby's heart rate and my contractions. Before I had a chance to ask him any questions, he was gone. The nurse said that he had a woman in active labor down the hall, but that my own doctor had just phoned the hospital and left a message that he was on his way.

As soon as the doctor left, John came back from the parking lot. The fresh air must have done him some good. He no longer had that Thousand-Mile Stare. He began joking with the nurse, telling her that this was going to be a do-it-yourself-grandson. The nurse loosened up to the point of cracking a smile.

I told John that the resident doctor didn't seem to think that having a baby four and a half weeks early was any cause for alarm. He had said that, just two nights earlier, he had delivered a baby born six weeks premature. The baby was perfectly healthy and had spent only one day in the incubator.

As I talked, the nurse was hooking up what is called a fetal monitor. It consists of two electrical units that are strapped to the abdomen, each about the size of a small portable radio, which in turn record their results on a cardiotocograph. When these instruments were attached, the nurse reminded me that I was to remain still. My contractions and the baby's heartbeat would be monitored by the units, and a needle would trace both the heart rate and the contractions in ink on graph paper. What they would be looking for on the graph was any sign that the baby was not getting enough oxygen.

I had been attached to the machine for about forty-five minutes when my own doctor arrived. Once I saw him I knew for sure that everything would be okay. There was no trace of panic in his face—not that it would show even if there was a problem. In fact the only time I had seen him with a worried expression was when I once told him that I had broken four basal thermometers. Three had flown out of my hand as I was shaking them down, and one broke when I ran it under hot water to make sure it was working. I think he was worried because he thought I would be a dangerous person to let loose around his lab and office equipment.

Before my doctor said anything to me he looked over at John, who was sitting in the chair clutching his wristwatch, ready to time my first contraction. He told John that he hadn't expected to see him anywhere near the labor room. John managed a laugh and said that he should have followed his gut instinct and put his coaching instructions on a taped cassette.

The doctor began studying the graph paper that was unrolling on the machine. After several minutes he told the nurse to take me off the monitor. I was not having any contractions. Then he turned toward me and said that I shouldn't worry about a thing. The baby had a good, steady heart rate, and even though I was early, the baby would be close to the size of a full-term—probably six pounds.

The most important thing to do now was to get a good night's rest. He said that, being only a fingertip dilated with no contractions, the chances were I wouldn't deliver for perhaps eight or nine hours. If I hadn't gone into active labor by midmorning, he would have to induce it, since once the amniotic sac ruptures, the baby is no longer protected from infection by the fluid. To avoid that risk, the baby should be delivered within forty-eight hours.

An hour after the doctor left, John was giving me a vocabulary test from a three-year-old *Reader's Digest* he found on the table. This was his idea of killing time. Suddenly I felt what I thought was a contraction. It began just as the Lamaze instructor had said it would—as mild menstrual cramping. The first and last part of the contraction was weak, and the middle was slightly stronger. The entire contraction lasted about forty-five seconds. In fact, once it was over, I thought that maybe it hadn't been a contraction at all. Since I didn't want to give John a false alarm, I said nothing, and we continued with the vocabulary test.

About fifteen minutes later, the same thing happened. This time I was sure it was a legitimate contraction. It was slightly stronger than the first one. When I told John that I was having my second contraction, he dropped the magazine to the floor, took off his watch, and wanted me to start the slow chest breathing. I reminded him of what our instructor had said: "Don't wear yourself out with the breathing exercises before you really need them."

When the third contraction came fifteen minutes later, I tried convincing John that I didn't need to do the breathing yet. But he refused to believe me. When he kept urging me to do the slow chest breathing I said, a little too loudly, "I don't need the breathing yet. And stop referring to my contractions as pains."

Just then the nurse walked in. She had heard the outburst and wanted to know whether my labor pains had begun. I decided not to correct her. Instead I told her that I had had three consecutive contractions, each of them lasting forty-five seconds. She looked over at John to confirm this, and then said that she would wait for the next one. But the next one came five minutes earlier than the other three. During the contraction, the nurse pressed her hand firmly on my abdomen. When the contraction was over, she said that she could tell by the tightening of the muscles that it had been very mild. But I told her that that contraction had *not* been mild. It had been about three times as strong as the others. She responded by narrowing her eyes and suggesting that I get some rest in order to save up for the real labor pains.

With those words there came a sound from down the hall that made my skin crawl. The nurse immediately took off in the direction of the wail. For the first few minutes neither John nor I could make out what the woman was howling. But it soon became apparent. She kept calling out her husband's name and repeating, "I can't take the pain any longer!" I assumed that the woman was in the pant-blow breathing stage. John assumed that she was a Lamaze school drop-out.

I had been in the labor room two and a half hours and still hadn't been able to get Patsy on the phone. Each time I tried, her line had been busy. But finally I got through.

"Patsy," I said, "I'm calling you from my bed in the labor room."

"Don't joke about that, Lizzy," she said.

I quickly told her that everything was okay. Both my doctor and the resident doctor agreed that the baby would be just fine. He would be about six pounds, and he had dropped into a good position for a normal delivery. Patsy was very quiet on the other end. Finally she began telling me that she knew that I would get through it without any problem. I would be just like those peasant women who have their babies in the field and are back working a few hours later. It was the first time in my entire pregnancy that Patsy left out the scare tactics.

I told Patsy that I had had a total of four contractions and that the last one had been so strong that I would probably have to start my breathing very soon. But Patsy didn't say anything more about the labor. She asked if we had decided between Colin and Christopher, and what did we think of the name Sean. I was about to tell her that on the way up to the labor room we had agreed on the name Christopher, but before I got that out, another contraction came. It was so strong I had to tell Patsy that I'd call her back. I hung up and did some sort of breathing exercise while rubbing my stomach in a circular motion, a Lamaze technique that was supposed to help relaxation. When the contraction was over I told John to get the nurse. I thought I was going to throw up.

While John was down the hall looking for her, I wobbled into the bathroom and did just that. A couple of minutes later they both came back. The nurse helped me out of the bathroom and into bed. No sooner had I gotten into bed than another contraction came. Again I did some sort of combination breathing that had nothing to do with what we had learned in class. The nurse told me that I was breathing too fast, and that I might hyperventilate. John wasn't saying anything about the breathing. He was too busy calling off how many seconds were left for the contraction. When the contraction peaked I started to do the circular rubbing, but the nurse removed my hands so that she could feel the strength of the contraction. When it was over she said that it was still quite mild and that I should really try to get some rest.

At that point John spoke up and said that the labor pains were coming every five to seven minutes and lasting for sixty seconds. But the nurse said that they still seemed mild and that it was possible that they would continue like that for the rest of the night.

When she said "the rest of the night" I looked over at John for him to do something—*anything*. He immediately came over to the bed and began rubbing the small of my back with his fist, another Lamaze technique helpful in relieving discomfort. He remained at my side for the next hour, timing the contractions while never missing a beat at the back rubbing.

By the time the hour was up, the contractions were coming every three to four minutes and lasting one minute. For each contraction I made up a different breathing exercise as I couldn't remember exactly which was which. All during this time, the woman in active labor down the hall was calling out, "Harry! I can't take the pain any longer!"

Listening to that woman, I wondered how much longer it would be before I began doing the same thing. If what the nurse had said was true—that I wasn't in real labor yet—what would it be like when I got to the real thing? Would I be able to take it?

After another half hour of intense contractions coupled with a string of "Harry! I can't take this any longer!" I told John to get the nurse. I wanted the strongest pain killer she had.

Just when John started toward the door, I heard the call for Harry suddenly stop. There was silence, then the wail of a newborn. It was amazing how that sudden shift from despair to joy helped me to forget, for a moment anyway, my own problems. I told John not to bother, and I laid back and waited for the next contraction. It came swift, fierce, and sure. With the pain of that contraction, I told John to get the nurse. This time I really did need a pain killer. Five minutes later I was given a shot of Phenergan, a muscle relaxant.

At some time after midnight, or about an hour and a half after the contractions first began, I felt an uncontrollable urge to push. Although all through the contractions I was never able to remember exactly which breathing exercise to use, I *did* remember what the instructor had said about pushing: "If you have the urge to push, first have either the doctor or the nurse examine you to make sure that you are fully dilated. Premature pushing will do no good and may cause damage to the cervix."

John called for the nurse, and within seconds she was back in the room. After examining me she announced in a startled tone that I was eight centimeters dilated—only two away from being able to push. After telling me to hold back on the pushing, she left to phone the doctor. He arrived in less than half an hour. It was probably the longest half hour of my life. John remained at the side of my bed, rubbing his fist against the small of my back and calling out how much time was left during each contraction. The contractions were now coming practically on top of one another. On the other side of the bed was the nurse—she was reminding me to pant-blow. I was so foggy I didn't know what I was doing.

The moment my doctor arrived he examined me

to find that I was now fully dilated. It was time to start pushing. This brought considerable relief from the pain. From then on, everything happened so fast I didn't even have time to worry about my next contraction. When my doctor left to scrub for the delivery, another nurse came in. There were now two nurses—one on either side of the bed. John had been relocated over to the chair where he continued telling me what a brave person I was.

The two nurses helped me into the Lamaze push position: semipropped with knees bent and hands under the knees, grasping the thighs. As each contraction began, I was instructed by both nurses at the same time to take a deep breath, hold it for as long as possible, and then push with all my strength for as long as I could.

Within five pushes the baby's head "crowned"— the top of the baby's head could be seen coming through the cervix. It was now time to be wheeled by stretcher into the delivery room.

In moments a stretcher was rolled in by the two nurses, who had changed quickly into green surgical gowns and masks. As soon as I was moved from my bed to the stretcher one of the nurses turned to John and handed him a surgical gown and mask. He stood up, slipped it on, and the nurse tied the strings in the back. Then she showed him how to adjust the mask. Seconds later, our convoy started off down the hall toward the delivery room.

As out of it as I was, it suddenly occurred to me that John was headed into the delivery room. This was someplace he had vowed *never* to enter. In fact John had stayed in the labor room, even though I told him twice that I would understand if and when he could no longer stand it. But maybe he sensed that I really didn't mean that. I needed him in that labor room. And now as the stretcher came to a rest beside a long table, I needed him more than ever. I was immediately lifted onto it. Bright lights were coming from all directions. My legs were strapped high in the air. I couldn't see John, but I felt his hands rubbing my temples and heard his voice, which he had now lowered about ten octaves for the sanctity of the delivery room.

At this point the doctor said that if I pushed down long and hard two more times the baby would be born. I did. And he was right. The next thing I heard was a faint cry. It wasn't a wail like Harry's baby had let out. Suddenly a surge of adrenaline shot through my body, removing all the pain and resulting in a euphoric numbness.

"Is my baby okay?" I didn't wait for the doctor to answer. "Are his toes okay?" I asked. I don't know why the toes took priority.

He didn't answer my question. All he said was, "Here's Christopher! What a beautiful nose." And the doctor held up the most beautiful five-pound, fourteen-and-a-half-ounce plucked chicken I had ever seen. Moments later the nurse placed him in my arms. His tiny features were all squashed. I didn't really notice the nose. His little head was slightly on the cone side, but he *was* beautiful. I had something in my arms I thought I'd never have. Something I used to go to bed at night crying for. This was the most magical moment in my life.

I don't know how long the nurse left him in my arms before she placed him in John's. It was probably a couple of minutes, but it seemed like a second. Yet it seemed like a lifetime.

"You're not afraid to hold him, are you?" the nurse said.

"Yes," John answered. "I am. But we really worked hard for this."

"John," the doctor said, "I thought the only way I'd ever see you in the delivery room would be blindfolded and gagged."

"I did too," John said. "I hardly knew I was coming in here. I think I was drugged."

Christopher was born at 3:04 in the morning. Less than an hour later, John and I were in a cheerful yellow and white room recapping the highlights of the birth. John kept going on about how he never thought he could have stayed for the birth, especially with those Lamaze slides still fresh in his memory. But when the nurse handed him the green gown and mask, it never entered his mind not to go in. It just seemed like the natural thing to do.

I kept telling John that if he hadn't been constantly at my side, calling off how much time was left for each contraction, I would have screamed a lot louder than Harry's wife down the hall. As it was, I ended up having the shot of Phenergan, the muscle relaxant. When those labor pains started coming on top of one another, my original intentions of having a drugless birth went right out the labor room door. I would have killed for even baby aspirin. But now it was all over. The only thing that mattered was that we had a beautiful, healthy baby who was now peacefully asleep in the nursery—or so I thought.

CHAPTER
12
Christopher

By the time daylight came, I was still wide awake and living off the high of Christopher's birth. John had left the hospital just before the first crack of light. He wanted to stay longer, but I told him that he may as well go home, get a few hours' rest, a shower, and a change of clothes so he would be fresh and alert when Christopher was brought to the room. I thought that would be sometime after breakfast. I didn't know how I was going to wait that long.

I wanted to phone my parents the moment we moved from the delivery room to my room, but John thought I should wait at least until seven. He said that it would frighten them if I called in the middle of the night. But it was now nearly seven. I couldn't wait another minute. I dialed the hospital operator and placed the long-distance call.

My father answered. Before I even said hello, I told him, "Congratulations. You have a grandson." Because he was half groggy from sleep, I had to repeat it a few times. Then he yelled for my mother to pick up the phone downstairs; within seconds everyone was on an extension.

There was dead silence as I told them that, even though the baby had come four and a half weeks early, he was just perfect. And that the labor lasted only four hours and John was with me the entire time. And that I couldn't have done it without him. I must have kept them on the phone an hour telling them all the details, even about Harry's wife screaming down the hall. And that John claimed Christopher looked just like his old Uncle Debe. But all of his kids looked like old Uncle Debe when they were first born.

After I reassured them that the baby was fine and I was too, my mother asked how long I would be in the hospital. I told her that I thought it would be no longer than three days, but I'd have to call her back later in the afternoon to confirm that. She said that she wanted to fly up the day before I came home so that she could get everything ready. Then the last thing she asked was whether I had the yellow or the pink nightgown on and whether I had remembered to pack the blue and white knit shawl.

Seconds after I hung up the phone rang. It was Patsy. She said that she had been trying to get through to me half the night, but the operator wouldn't put the call through until eight. I told her that I was just about to phone to tell her that everything was just perfect. Then I began telling her basically the same things I had told my family. But I added a few of the gruesome birth details because I felt that was what she was dying to know. I had just gotten to the part about the final push when I heard the sound of babies crying and then saw a few of them being wheeled past my room to their mothers' rooms. I told Patsy that the babies were coming around and I would call her as soon as I fed Christopher. I was so excited I dropped the phone.

There must have been half a dozen babies pushed in their plastic bassinets past my open door. I was trying to remember what color Christopher's hair was when I heard a very loud cry—it must have been Harry's baby. Or maybe it was my baby and he was hungry. I had planned on breast feeding and I was a little nervous thinking that for some reason I might not be able to.

Fifteen minutes had passed since I had first seen the babies being taken down the corridor to their mothers. I began to wonder where Christopher was. Then I thought that perhaps because he was only five hours old they were going to let him sleep a little longer. Just then a nurse came in to take my temperature. She asked why I hadn't touched my breakfast tray. I told her I would get to it after I had fed my baby. And where was my baby?

She looked a little surprised and asked, "Hasn't your pediatrician been in to see you yet?"

"Pediatrician," I said. "No. Why?" I was suddenly confused.

But she didn't say anything more than, "I'll go see where he is." She left without even taking my temperature.

My first reaction was near panic. But then I realized that it was probably just a hospital policy: he probably wanted to come around and talk to me about breast feeding first. That was it, I was sure. But I still didn't think it was necessary for the nurse to keep me hanging.

I must have waited there another ten minutes. It seemed like an eternity. All was quiet in the hall now. There were no bassinets being rolled by the open door. Finally, when it was obvious that all the babies were now feeding with their mothers, I pushed the hospital call button. There was no response for a moment, but then there was a soft knock on the half-open door, and the pediatrician came in.

I was hoping to see a smile on his face, but he looked very serious. I couldn't quite understand why. After all, I had just given birth to a very beautiful baby. He spoke softly and said, "Mrs. Fuller, I have just come from seeing your baby."

All I did was nod my head. I suddenly found myself afraid to speak.

"There is some problem with Christopher," he said. "But I'm sure we'll be able to handle it."

"Problem?" I said.

"There's a condition called Hyaline Membrane Disease," he said. "It sometimes comes with premature development of the lungs. There is some respiratory distress, but he is getting plenty of oxygen and we're monitoring him carefully."

The impact of what he was saying would not register. I could hardly take in his words. I didn't know how to respond. He went on to tell me that the blood oxygen was holding up well, that he was in the Intensive Care Unit, and that he was receiving the best kind of care and treatment. But it would take the next twelve to twenty-four hours to see how he would respond to it. I would be allowed to go down to Intensive Care in a wheelchair, but he wanted to let me know what to expect, and not to be frightened by the apparatus temporarily hooked up to the baby: intravenous fluids, heart monitor, oxygen hood, oxygen monitor, and other equipment.

All I wanted to do was see my baby. I knew I couldn't hold him, but at least I could see him. The nurse brought in a special gown and a wheelchair, and in moments I was pushed into the Intensive Care Unit. I could hardly see the baby in the isolette for all the tubes and equipment, but there he was, breathing fitfully, eyes closed—and beautiful. I found myself half wanting to rip off the tubes and hold him to me. Instead, I sat as close as I could to the isolette and watched, praying with every breath he took. Beside me was the heart monitor, a televisionlike screen with a bright green bouncing ball moving endlessly across the screen in rhythm with his fast-beating heart. The sound was amplified and in synchronization with the ball on the screen. It was steady, thank God. His tiny chest was gulping air much too fast, I thought, rising and falling spasmodically.

I gripped the arms of the wheelchair until my knuckles were white, watching and praying. Above the oxygen hood was a meter. The nurse explained that it showed the percentage of oxygen being pumped into the chamber. It read "40" on the small digital screen; this meant 40 percent oxygen. They were careful not to give too much; it could cause blindness. They told me that they hoped to reduce the amount of oxygen gradually to a normal level—22 or 24 percent. But it would be a slow process. They had already taken three chest X-rays, and were treating him with ampicillin in case pneumonia had developed.

I must have been sitting there, motionless, for an hour. The nurses kept giving me words of encouragement as I watched. Then John came in, not having known the baby's condition until he had reached the hospital. He was terribly upset, I could tell, but he was trying to hide it, trying to reassure me, saying that the doctor had told him about the blood oxygen level, which he had said was good in spite of the problem. Together we sat there, saying little, staring into the plexiglass cage, terrified. At one point, a warning light flashed on the instrument panel and a buzzer sounded, frightening and alarming us. But the nurse quickly assured us that all was well—it was just a quirk of the machine. We finally went back to my room, numb with suspense.

From then on, the waiting was almost unbearable. I spent most of my time in the Intensive Care Unit, only returning to my room to pick at some food and try to sleep. Each time, I checked the oxygen percentage indicator—praying that they would be able to reduce it. By Sunday, the third day after the birth, it was down to thirty-five. Then thirty. Then twenty-eight. Only a few more points to reach normal room oxygen. By Monday, it was down to regular room oxygen; Christopher could breathe normally at last. He was moved from Intensive Care into a regular isolette, although the ampicillin treatment was continued for a short while thereafter.

On the fifth day after Christopher's birth his bassinet was wheeled into my room, where it remained the entire day and night. During that first day I nursed him, changed him, held him; I was completely in charge of his every need. The only time he left my arms was when the nurse put him back into his bassinet so that I could eat and sleep. I suddenly felt very much the same as I had when I was five years old taking care of my Tiny Tears doll.

Early the following morning, the pediatrician came to say goodbye. He reminded me once again that Christopher was leaving the hospital with a clean bill of health. There would be *no* aftereffects. Once he was over it, he was over it.

As I dressed Christopher in his little blue going-home suit, I couldn't help thinking that this marked the beginning of a new life, not only for Christopher, but also for John and me. I had no idea how this new beginning would change our lives. That no longer seemed important. All my past fears of losing self-identity or turning into Christopher's personal robot had vanished completely during those long days in the Intensive Care Unit, when I watched him gasp for each breath as if it were his last. It was at that time I realized just what really mattered in life. However, as I slipped Christopher's matching blue bonnet onto his tiny head, I did wonder if John and I would be able to continue to travel with Christopher tagging along.

Now, with Christopher well, I felt as if I could accomplish anything. In spite of the nursery routine, which I was looking forward to, I would still have extra time, especially since I no longer had to waste countless hours poring over temperature charts and crying over the phone to Patsy, Donna, my doctor, or to anyone who would listen. That alone had wasted more productive man hours than I cared to count. But on the other hand, as Patsy pointed out the first time she saw Christopher through the nursery window, maybe all that seemingly wasted time hadn't been spent in vain. She said that if I hadn't been so determined to have a baby, I probably would have given up after that first miscarriage. And had I done that, I wouldn't be wrapping Christopher in in his blue and white knit shawl now.

John, Christopher, and I left the hospital just before noon. On the parkway John drove as if he were maneuvering the royal coach through a crowded procession. I sat in the back seat clutching Christopher, half tempted to give the smug royal wave out the back window. As we made the final turn into our driveway, no heralds or beefeaters were on hand to greet us. But my mother was there. Her face said what no amount of pomp and circumstance could express. As I placed Christopher in her greedy outstretched arms, no words were spoken. It was too sacred an event. But there were tears—tears that said miracles can still happen if you wait long enough.

AFTERWORD

No one likes to admit an abrupt about-face. I, however, am forced to. All through Elizabeth's turmoil in yearning for an offspring, I was a reluctant dragon, at one moment hoping that the whole process would really fail; at another, hoping that her wish would come true. I had had three children from former marriages, the youngest of whom was just starting college when Project Christopher was in process. The thought of facing midnight feedings, Pampers, jammed rubber nipples that wouldn't let the milk through, unmotivated wailing, Cub Scouts, Little League, and PTA meetings was enough to give me nightmares.

But from the moment we brought Christopher

165

home from the hospital, something happened. All those concerns suddenly vacated my mind. I don't exactly know what it was that did it. Maybe it was those tiny toes, smaller than spring peas in a pod. Or fingernails that looked like the smallest pearl on a string. Or eyes of the deepest blue a painter could mix. And when the first series of smiles came in the third month, I was sure they must have been computer-enhanced.

The whole turnabout from slightly sullen acquiescence to beamish paternal pride would not be so marked if it were not for my slide into downright sloppy sentimentality. I make excuses to wake him up at times, just to look at him. I pick him up and walk him around the room when there is absolutely no reason for it. I remind Elizabeth it's my turn to change his diaper. I even tape-record his chortling in the hopes of catching the first word that is gummed out of his toothless mouth, although I'm sure he'll have teeth when this happens.

I have to admit to a certain sense of pride in admitting how wrong I was in resisting the idea of a baby. It takes a big man to admit this. In spite of my resistance, Elizabeth was right all along. A baby brings a hefty measure of joy and fulfillment, and there's only one condition where I have already been forced to put my foot down: Christopher can have plenty of friends and fawning relatives. But a brother or sister? I'm afraid not. I've made my last about-face.

John G. Fuller
Westport, Connecticut
September 1982

GLOSSARY

ADHESIONS: scar tissue that forms on organs, binding them together. This usually happens after an operation or an infection.

AID: abbreviation for artificial insemination using the sperm of an anonymous donor

AIH: abbreviation for artificial insemination using the sperm of the husband

AMNIOCENTESIS: procedure in which amniotic fluid is withdrawn from the amniotic sac for chromosomal analysis in the fourteenth to twentieth week of pregnancy

ANNOVULATION: lack of ovulation

BASAL BODY TEMPERATURE: temperature taken first thing after waking

CERVIX: the neck of the uterus

CHROMOSOME: a unit of genetic material containing the DNA "blueprint" for each individual. The forty-six chromosomes are in the nucleus of every cell in the body, except for the sperm and egg, each containing twenty-three. When a sperm fertilizes an egg, the embryo receives a total of forty-six chromosomes, half from each parent.

CLOMIPHENE CITRATE: also called Clomid. This drug stimulates the pituitary gland to stimulate in turn the ovaries to release an egg.

CORPUS LUTEUM: a yellow mass that forms on the surface of the ovaries at the time of ovulation. It is this yellow mass that is responsible for the production of the hormone progesterone.

DOPPLER ULTRA-SOUND: a special machine used to detect the fetal heartbeat as early as the twelfth week of pregnancy

ENDOMETRIOSIS: a condition that occurs when part of the normal uterine lining appears outside the uterus in areas such as the tubes, ovaries, or the surface of the abdominal cavity

ENDOMETRIUM: the lining of the uterus

ESTROGEN: a hormone produced by the ovaries. Estrogen is needed for menstruation, sex development, and pregnancy.

FALLOPIAN TUBE: a narrow tube connecting the ovary and the uterus, through which the egg travels. It is about four inches long. There are two Fallopian tubes—one on each side of the uterus.

FERTILITY: the ability to have a child

FERTILITY DRUG: a drug that either directly or indirectly stimulates the ovaries to release one or more eggs

FERTILIZATION: the moment the sperm joins the egg

FIBROIDS: nonmalignant tumors of the uterus

FOLLICLE-STIMULATING HORMONE (FSH): FSH is responsible for stimulating the egg inside the ovary to ripen, mature, and then emerge from the surface of the ovary.

GONORRHEA: a venereal disease. Left untreated, it could spread throughout the reproductive tract, destroying the tubes.

HYSTEROSALPINGOGRAM: an X-ray of the uterus and Fallopian tubes after a radiopaque dye is injected through the cervix. If the dye spills through the tubes this indicates that the tubes are not blocked.

IMPLANTATION: when the fertilized egg attaches itself to the wall of the uterus

IMPOTENCE: failure to achieve an erection

IUD (INTRAUTERINE DEVICE): a coil-type contraceptive device that is placed by a physician into the uterus to interfere with implantation of the fertilized egg

KARYOTYPE: a display of 23 chromosomes that have been photographed, enlarged, cut individually, and arranged on paper

LAMAZE: prepared childbirth developed by the French doctor Ferdinand Lamaze. The purpose of the course is to educate couples as to exactly what is happening during each stage of labor so that the couples can work positively with the labor, keeping the discomfort and drugs down to a minimum.

LAPAROSCOPY: a surgical operation in which a thin telescopelike instrument equipped with light and lens is inserted through the navel to examine the Fallopian tubes and other pelvic organs

LUTEINIZING HORMONE (LH): a hormone released by the pituitary; it is responsible for stimulating the egg inside the ovary to ripen and mature

MISCARRIAGE: loss of the fetus before it is able to survive outside the uterus

MOTILITY: action of normal forward-moving sperm

OVARY: the female sex gland that secretes the egg cells. There are two ovaries—one on each side of the uterus.

PELVIC INFLAMMATORY DISEASE, OR P.I.D.: infection involving the female reproductive organs that could lead to damage of the Fallopian tubes

PHENERGAN: a muscle relaxant

PITUITARY: a gland that sits at the base of the brain. It secretes the hormones necessary for growth, puberty, and pregnancy.

POSTCOITAL: a procedure in which a sample of cervical mucous is examined under a microscope. A normal test would reveal the cervical mucous to be thin, clear, watery, and stretchable with an abundance of motile sperm penetrating it.

PROGESTERONE: often called the hormone of pregnancy. It is secreted by the corpus luteum of the ovary. In pregnancy it is produced by the placenta.

SEMEN ANALYSIS: the microscopic study of sperm ejaculated within two to four hours to determine the number of sperm per cubic centimeter, their shape and size, along with their ability to move in a forward motion

SPONTANEOUS ABORTION: loss of fetus within the first twelve weeks of pregnancy

TEMPERATURE CHARTS: a daily record of the early-morning temperature plotted during the entire monthly cycle in order to determine ovulation, which would be indicated by a mid-cycle temperature drop of half to one degree, followed by a sharp rise

VARICOCELE: a varicose vein in the scrotum, believed to be responsible for about 40 percent of male infertility

BIBLIOGRAPHY

Amelard, M.D., Richard. *Infertility in Men*. Philadelphia: F. A. Davis, 1966.

Barker, Dr. Graham H. *Your Search for Fertility*. New York: William Morrow, 1981.

Behrman, M.D., Samuel and Robert W. Kistner, M.D. *Progress in Infertility*. Boston: Little, Brown, 1968.

Bing, Elizabeth and Libby Colman. *Having a Baby After Thirty*. New York: Bantam, 1980.

Blais, Madeline. *They Say You Can't Have a Baby*. New York: W. W. Norton, 1979.

Brewer, Gail Sforza and Janice Presser Greene. *Right from the Start*. Emmaus, Pa.: Rodale Press, 1981.

172

Brody, Jane. "Fetal Health." *New York Times.* 16 February 1982.

Brozan, Nadine. "Infertility: Couples' Reactions." *New York Times.* 26 July 1982.

Chesler, Phyllis. *With Child.* New York: Thomas Y. Crowell, 1979.

Decker, M.D., Albert and Suzanne Loebl. *Why Can't We Have a Baby?* New York: Dial, 1978.

Dullea, Georgia. "Women Reconsider Childbearing Over 30." *New York Times.* 25 February 1982.

Harrison, Mary. *Infertility.* Boston: Houghton Mifflin, 1977.

Hinds, Michael deCourcy. "FDA May Warn on Drugs in Pregnancy." *New York Times.* 28 August 1982.

Howard, Jr., M.D., James T. and Dodi Schultz. *We Want to Have a Baby.* New York: E. P. Dutton, 1979.

Kaufman, M.D., Sherwin A. *From a Gynecologist's Notebook.* New York: Stein and Day, 1974.

Kaufman, M.D., Sherwin A. *You Can Have a Baby.* Nashville: Thomas Nelson, 1978.

Lawson, Patricia and Fredda Simon. *Childbirth Preparation Manual.* Waban, MA: Lawson/Simon, 1975.

McCauley, Carole Spearin. *Pregnancy After 35.* New York: Pocket Books, 1976.

Menning, Barbara Eck. *Infertility.* Englewood Cliffs, NJ: Prentice-Hall, 1977.

Nilsson, Lennart. *A Child Is Born.* New York: Dell, 1965.

Queenan, M.D., John T., ed. *A New Life.* New York: Van Nostrand Reinhold, 1979.

Silber, M.D., Sherman J. *How to Get Pregnant.* New York: Scribner's, 1980.

Span, Paula. "Infertility." *Glamour* magazine. December 1981.

Stangel, M.D., John J. *Fertility and Conception.* New York: Paddington Press, 1979.

Tucker, Tarvez with Elizabeth Bing. *Prepared Childbirth.* Wayne, PA: Banbury Books, 1975.

Wachstein, Alison Ehrlich. *Pregnant Moments.* New York: Morgan and Morgan, 1979.

Webster, Bayard. "Study Shows Female Fertility Drops Sharply After Age of 30." *New York Times.* 18 February 1982.